Developmental Motor
Speech Disorders

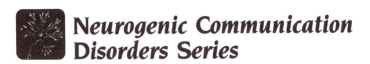

Neurogenic Communication Disorders Series

SERIES EDITOR
Leonard L. LaPointe, Ph.D.

Developmental Motor Speech Disorders
Michael A. Crary

Cognitive-Communicative Deficits Following Traumatic Brain Injury: Functional Approaches
Leila L. Hartley

Pediatric Traumatic Brain Injury: Implementing a Proactive Response
Jean L.Blosser and Roberta DePompei

Developmental Motor Speech Disorders

Michael A. Crary, Ph.D.

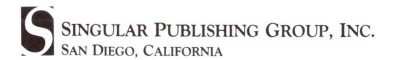

SINGULAR PUBLISHING GROUP, INC.
SAN DIEGO, CALIFORNIA

Published by Singular Publishing Group, Inc.
4284 41st Street
San Diego, California 92105-1197

©1993 by Singular Publishing Group, Inc.

Typeset in 10.5/12 Goudy Oldstyle by CFW Graphics
Printed in the United States of America by BookCrafters

Library of Congress Cataloging-in-Publication Data

Crary, Michael A., 1952–
    Developmental motor speech disorders / Michael A. Crary.
        p.   cm.
    Includes bibliographical references and index.
    ISBN 1-879105-92-6
    1. Articulation disorders in children.   2. Apraxia.   I. Title.
    [DNLM: 1. Speech Disorders—physiopathology.   2. Language
    Development Disorders—diagnosis.   3. Motor Skills—physiology.   WL
    340 C893d 1993]
RJ496.S7C74   1993
618.92′8552—dc20
DNLM/DLC
for Library of Congress   93-3711
                                                                      CIP

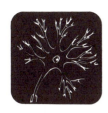

Contents

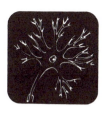

Foreword

The brain is a marvelous thing. It has been called the only human organ capable of studying itself. While the metaphoric heart has been rhapsodized in song and sonnet much more frequently, the brain and its peculiar music has met increasing attention, not only popularly, but notably from researchers, scholars, educators, and clinicians who must deal with attempts to understand it. In fact, in the United States, the commitment to understanding the brain and its disorders has been reflected in the highest policy levels of the government, and the White House Office of Science and Technology Policy focused this attention in a report entitled "Maximizing Human Potential: Decade of the Brain 1990–2000."

When the human nervous system goes awry, the cost is enormous. Direct and indirect economic impact of brain disorders in the United States has been estimated to be over 400 billion dollars. It is impossible to measure the toll that brain disorders extract in terms of human agony from victims and their families. Each disruption of delicate neural balance can cause problems in moving, sensing, eating, thinking, and a rich array of human behaviors. Certainly not the least of these are those unique human attributes involved in communication. To speak, to understand, to write, to read, to remember, to create, to calculate, to plan, to reason . . . and myriad other cognitive and communicative acts are the sparks and essence of human interaction. When they are lost or impaired, isolation can result or, at the very least, quality of life can be compromised. This series is about the many conditions that arise from brain or nervous system damage that can affect these human cognitive and communicative functions. But it is not only an attempt to understand the disruption and negative effects of neurogenic disorders. As well, the authors in this series will show that there is a positive side. Rehabilitation, relearning, intervention, recovery, adjustment, acceptance, and reintegration are the rewards to be extracted from challenge. There will be no shortage of these features in this series. Frustrations and barriers can be redeemed by recovery and small victories. The works in this Singular Series on Neurogenic Communication Disorders will address both the obstacles and the triumphs.

The first book in this series addresses the theme of motor speech disorders in children. This is a puzzling and controversial topic that has spawned debate and confusion. Michael Crary brings a background of experience and insight to the topic and has created a work that will benefit not only scholars and students who wish to learn about or gain a new perspective on the disorders, but clinicians who must meet the daily challenges of working with these children and their families.

Leonard L. LaPointe, Ph.D.
Series Editor

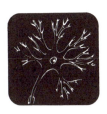

Preface

All of us have come across children with severe speech disorders in our clinical work. Fortunately, for them and for us, these encounters do not dominate clinical practice. I have heard repeatedly from clinicians that they see two or three such children unless they are in settings prone to attract especially severe problems. Although the frequency of these problems is not staggering, the severity is. Most clinicians will admit that these cases do dominate their available time and resources. Most clinicians wish that they had more time and resources to devote to these children.

Children with severe speech production deficits in the absence of other, more general problems, may be considered to reflect deviant motor speech control. Historically, the label of apraxia of speech (or one of its variants) has been used, often indiscriminately, to describe such problems. This label has been applied, appropriately or inappropriately, to a variety of problems, typically due to the perception of some type of motor speech deficit by the examining clinician. The disparity among applications of this label has been a source of confusion and controversy for years. Neither clinicians nor researchers, despite substantial effort and discussion, have been able to negotiate an agreeable compromise to this controversy. Yet, they remain—these children who struggle to produce even the simplest of communications.

Over 15 years ago, I became interested in apraxia of speech, first, as an academic endeavor and, later, after meeting several children so diagnosed, as a clinical challenge. *Developmental Motor Speech Disorders* is an accumulation of what I have learned from these children during the last 15 years. There have been many children, all different in their own way. Some improved, some did not, at least not as a result of my efforts. All were teachers as much as they were learners. I have tried to be honest in reporting what I have learned. In many instances questions prevailed over answers. Many unanswered questions remain. Perhaps the single most important aspect of developmental motor speech disorders that I would like to share is that of perspective. This theme is revisited again and again throughout this book. No single developmental motor speech disorder exists. Rather, a group of problems may be encountered with some common characteristics, but with many differentiating features.

Envision this book in three sections. The initial section (Chapters 1, 2, and 3) attempts to lay the theoretical groundwork for a motolinguistic model of developmental motor speech disorders. The second section (Chapters 4, 5, 6, and 7) considers characteristics and abilities of children with developmental motor speech disorders. The final section (Chapters 8 and 9) directly addresses the clinical management of such problems with practical suggestions for assessment and intervention strategies. *Developmental Motor Speech Disorders* was not written for any specific market audience. Rather, it was written in attempt to synthesize available information, present new or little known information, and suggest assessment and intervention strategies. Academicians and researchers will find many bones to pick. This is encouraged. Students may find a mix of ideas to be discussed, digested, or dismantled. Most importantly, clinicians will find suggestions that may be applied systematically to children who need extra help. Do not accept them without question. The sauce of experience will enhance any dish.

It is important to acknowledge those whose names do not appear on any title page. First, thanks to the many children and parents who allowed me to "try" things that I could not prove. They are the ghost writers. My family deserves a special award for tolerating me during this adventure. My natural idiosyncracies make life with me tough enough. Thanks for going the extra mile. Cudos to Dr. L. L. LaPointe (L^3) who took a dry martini, appreciated only by a select few, and turned it into a margarita that may be enjoyed by a variety of readers. Blessings to Marie Linvill who knew just the right time to call with a push, a laugh, or the perfect words of encouragement. My sincere appreciation to Sandy Doyle and to Mr. Buffett, Mr. Clapton, and Mr. Cale for getting me through the tedium of copy editing. Last, but not least, gratitude to my old friend Sadanand Singh who gave me the chance to tell this story.

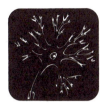 P R O L O G U E

A Human Perspective

An Inquiry

Dear Doctor,

I am interested in information on developmental apraxia of speech. My son, age 7, has just completed kindergarten. Because of his speech and motor delays I held him back an extra year in preschool. If it were not for the efforts of an elementary school principal he would be in a class for the retarded. He said hardly anything until a speech therapist used an electric toothbrush with him at age six. He still has no significant handwriting. After a year the speech therapist became frustrated when his one-word use did not become two and put all of her efforts into a talking computer instead. He never really took to it and seldom turns to it. He now has a three-word phrase on occasion but has not made any big leaps. It is becoming very hard to continue to support his intellect with so little to work with. IQ tests that use speech don't show his true ability. His current speech therapist uses the same old methods and he does respond at times but there is little carryover. He also sees a physical therapist who has him on her computer and her goals make things seem pretty bleak. I am afraid of the first grade and for his future. There really does seem to be a light in his eyes and actions that just can't be tapped yet. I would appreciate any advice or help that you could offer.

Sincerely,

A Concerned Mom

Reading letters like this has become an all too familiar experience for many clinicians. It's refrain contains elements common to many communicative problems: a severe speech problem with concomitant motor limitations, delayed onset of speech, academic failure, frustrated therapists, parents who would do anything to help a child "who would be normal if only he could talk." Fortunately, not every child who requires speech-language therapy demonstrates such a severe impairment. Unfortunately, the children who fit this scenario are the most challenging for parents and professionals and at the greatest risk for failure in other areas. These children typically present a complex, multifactorial problem. Yet, a single attribute all too frequently becomes the focus for the clinical diagnosis and the intervention strategy—the motor component.

No one knows exactly how many children demonstrate disorders of speech production. According to a fact sheet provided by the American Speech-Language-Hearing Association, an estimated 2.6 million Americans suffer from speech or language disorders. This estimate includes more than 50% of all handicapped children enrolled in Head Start programs. Articulation disorders account for nearly 60% of all speech and language disorders. What percentage of these individuals demonstrate articulation disorders related to motor limitations? Again, no one knows. Some believe that every child with an articulation disorder has some degree of motor speech impairment. Others reject the notion of motor-based articulation problems in children altogether except in cases where an overt sensorimotor problem suggests the diagnosis of dysarthria. In reality, the true picture probably lies somewhere between these philosophical extremes. There are some children who demonstrate severe deficits in speech articulation abilities secondary to developmental motor speech limitations. The true clinical challenge is to identify these children accurately and to structure intervention programs that will maximize their potential for improved speech and minimize the negative influence that impaired speech may have on other aspects of their development.

How Shall a Thing Be Called?

The most common label applied to children demonstrating a speech disorder suspected to be related to sensorimotor deficits is some variant of the term "apraxia," including developmental apraxia of speech, developmental verbal apraxia, developmental verbal dyspraxia, developmental articulatory apraxia, and so on. Clinicians may reserve the use of such terms for their most perplexing and difficult cases. Teachers come to understand the term as indicating limited progress and invasion of the speech disorder into other areas of academic performance. Parents learn to fear the term as one that limits the outlook for a child who otherwise seems normal and functional.

It is, however, most unfortunate that these labels are used with little understanding of the underlying problems faced by the child. It is unlikely that all children labeled as "apraxic" actually demonstrate a strong component of apraxia. Some may demonstrate a degree of apraxic component; others may demonstrate motor deficits more appropriately identified as dysarthria. Clinicians are not the villain in this situation. Ignorance is. Not individual ignorance, but generalized lack of specific knowledge. With limited specific knowledge, we face a lack of clinical and theoretical perspective.

A Starting Point

The intent in writing the following chapters is to provide a starting point for the development of improved clinical intervention in cases of articulation disorders that are suspected to result from motor dysfunction. The general orientation is to recognize that there are multiple forms of motor deficits that may contribute to developmental speech disorders. Rather than taking a label-specific approach to assessment and treatment, a model is offered from which to approach a group of developmental motor speech disorders. Patterns of performance on motor, motor speech, and speech tasks are used to profile the child with a developmental motor speech disorder. Resulting performance profiles may be used as a basis for inferring underlying deficits, but, more importantly, for planning appropriate intervention.

To begin, Chapter 1 presents an historical perspective focusing on traditional views of developmental dysarthria and apraxia of speech. A neurolinguistic perspective is offered in Chapter 2 in which the underpinnings of an explanatory model are reviewed. This chapter portrays the potential for multiple, interactive problems to exist in the child with a developmental motor speech disorder. A motolinguistic model is presented in Chapter 3. Based on the neurolinguistic principles offered in Chapter 2, the model presents a simplified conceptualization of a continuum of motor and language behaviors. Basic definitions and expected performance profiles are delineated in consideration of this model. Chapters 4 through 7 present performance characteristics of the child with a developmental motor speech disorder. Most of this information is based on work in the area of apraxia of speech, but when possible interpretations relevant to dysarthria are offered. Finally, Chapters 8 and 9 offer strategies for clinical assessment of and intervention for the child with a developmental motor speech disorder. These strategies are consistent with the motolinguistic model in consideration of both the child's abilities and the properties of clinical tools.

Clay Versus Stone

One of the delightful things about ideas is that they change. The content of the following chapters is scribbled in clay not etched in stone. Many of these ideas will and should be challenged. Suggested strategies should be tried, adopted when successful, and modified when unsuccessful. Beliefs should be shaken, and ultimately, new ideas should be born. There is a lot we don't know about children with developmental motor speech disorders. If we do not suggest, experiment, criticize, and change, the ultimate losers will be the children.

A *Response*

Dear Concerned Mom,

I share your frustration and concerns regarding your son. Unfortunately, there is much we do not know about children accused of demonstrating developmental apraxia of speech. It is not possible for me to offer specific advice to you without a thorough evaluation, but I will suggest some basic guidelines that you may want to review with the speech pathologist and the physical therapist as well as educational specialists in your area. What are the properties of his motor and speech deficits? Does he show a motor weakness, incoordination, other limitations? Is there any apparent relationship between the motor and speech problems? Do they share similar characteristics? How does your son communicate? What are his strengths and weaknesses in day-to-day communication? Do you have a grasp on his language processing abilities? What academic areas are his strengths? Why does he fail in other areas? And, finally, which therapeutic and academic strategies have shown the most promise and which have shown the least? The answers to these and other questions may help to put a focus on your son's difficulties and suggest a positive direction for the future.

In closing I would encourage you and your son's therapists not to give in to frustration. Keep trying. Focus on the child and not the label. There are few hard and fast answers at this time, but don't stop asking the questions.

Sincerely,

A Concerned Clinician

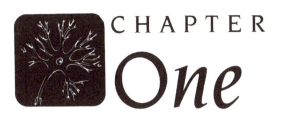

CHAPTER
One

An Historical Perspective

Directions and Misdirections

All children with speech production deficits are not the same. Although this sounds like a truism, all clinicians may not realize the extent of this assertion. We tend to recognize general "subtypes" of communicative impairments in children, but often fail to acknowledge the extensive variability within a given subtype when evaluating and treating these problems. We speculate and sometimes attempt to prove that different etiologies exist for communicative deficits but often are unable to incorporate such information in a clinically useful manner. We believe in the influence of strengths and/or impairments of various information processing systems underlying the overt characteristics of communicative deficits; however, many of our clinical protocols for evaluation and treatment focus on description of overt signs and symptoms and ignore potential underlying processing strategies. A comprehensive clinical approach should include description of overt symptoms, investigation of contributing etiologies, and evaluation of strengths and weaknesses of other influences such as underlying cognitive processes. By focusing on only one or two aspects of the clinical profile we may provide misdirected treatment.

A Common Example

The following example serves to illustrate the preceding point. A patient enters a physician's office complaining of generalized fatigue with intermittent respiratory difficulty. A history of recent weight loss is reported. On examination the physician finds no focal deficits. At this point in time the physician is left without a diagnosis and is unable to recommend appropriate treatment. This patient could have a relatively benign problem such as a cold or a more serious problem such as flu or pneumonia. This patient could have a neuromotor disease that is restricting ability to breathe. More than one factor may be contributing to this patient's overt symptoms. To identify the nature of the problem and hence offer effective treatment, the physician must look at the underlying cause(s) of the overt signs and symptoms. Until this is completed, a true understanding of the problem is lacking and the most effective treatment may be delayed or not provided.

Closer to Home

The theme of this scenario is all too common in the realm of communicative disorders. A 4-year-old child is brought to a speech-language pathologist for consultation. This child was observed to begin speaking later than his parents would have expected and/or liked. The parents feel the child is clumsy compared to his brothers and sisters. The child is not a good eater—very picky and tends to avoid certain types of food. Above all, the child's speech is difficult to understand, and the parents feel that he doesn't form good sentences. However, they report that he seems to understand most of what is said to him and they do not suspect any difficulty with his hearing. The pediatrician can find no structural or functional deficits including any signs of abnormal neurological function. This is a common clinical puzzle faced by the speech-language pathologist. We can describe the child's speech production errors and other aspects of language ability in reference to patterns of errors and/or developmentally based performance levels and develop a treatment based on the overt characteristics. In some cases, this may be a successful approach. If we can identify treatable causative factors (etiology), we may be able to indicate successful treatment of a different nature. Unfortunately, etiology is not always apparent, and causative factors typically do not offer themselves for easy identification. We might attempt some detective work to identify sources of difficulty that might contribute to the overt symptoms and treat what we believe may be underlying deficits. Unfortunately, the extent of our knowledge about the processes underlying many communicative disorders is limited. Few clinical procedures are available for evaluation or treatment of potential processes underlying the gamut of speech and language problems. These practical clinical limitations apply to many types of communicative disorders.

The Historical Role of Motor Problems

One issue that persists regarding children with severe deficits of speech production concerns the role of underlying motor/motor speech limitations in the disordered pattern. Significant controversy has simmered for years on the influence of motor speech deficits in children with severe articulation/phonologic problems. At least two types of motor speech explanations have been advanced to account for severe speech production disorders in children. The more notorious concept is that of apraxia or dyspraxia of speech. The more accepted concept is that of dysarthria secondary to neuromotor dysfunction. Developmental dysarthria typically is ascribed to children who demonstrate a generalized neuromuscular impairment such as that seen in the various forms of cerebral palsy. There is, however, ample historical description of developmental dysarthrias focal to the speech production mechanism in the absence of overt neuromuscular signs in other areas of the body. Although the concept of apraxia of speech has been both embraced and assaulted by clinicians and researchers for years, the concept of an isolated developmental dysarthria has been ignored by most. It is quite likely that many researchers and clinicians have lumped children with dysarthria and apraxia into one group. The history of our approach to these children has been a tortuous road influenced by the way we describe overt characteristics, presumptions about etiologies, and impressions about motoric and linguistic processes that might be impaired and/or preserved in such children. In the hope of developing an infrastructure for a better understanding of these communicative disorders, the following pages present an historical synopsis of clinical research of developmental dysarthria and apraxia of speech.

Early Perspectives from the British

In the early 1950s Muriel Morley and her colleagues (Morley, Court, & Miller, 1954) offered what they called a "simplified classification of speech disorders . . . . conceived within the framework of accepted neurological terminology" (p. 8). These clinical investigators believed that such a classification system was important in that "our continuing uncertainty about many of the cerebral processes involved in speech make it also a significant diagnostic problem for the family doctor and specialist" (Morley, Court, Miller, & Garside, 1955, p. 463). Their classification system included five broad diagnostic categories: disorders arising from deafness, aphasia, dysarthria, dyslalia, and stammering. Table 1–1 summarizes their classification system as presented in 1955. Of particular interest are the subcategories of dysarthria and aphasia and the category of dyslalia.

Morley, Court, and Miller (1954) defined dysarthria as "slow and clumsy articulation arising from dysfunction of the muscles used in speech" (p. 8). They pointed out the well known association with cerebral palsy, but recognized a group of children that present dysarthria as the "only disorder without detectible neurologic abnormality in any other part of the body" (p. 8). They described four patterns of developmental dysarthria: (1) dysarthria with clumsy movements of the lip, tongue, and palate; (2) dysarthria with clumsy

Table 1–1. Classification of speech disorders by Morley, Court, Miller, and Garside (1955).

Disorders Arising from Deafness
1. Congenital nerve deafness
    a. across all frequencies
    b. selective at high frequencies
2. Acquired nerve deafness

Aphasia
1. Developmental aphasia
    a. mainly receptive
        1. auditory imperception
        2. alexia
    b. mainly expressive
2. Acquired aphasia
3. Aphasia associated with general mental deficiency

Dysarthria
1. Anatomic defects including cleft palate
2. Dysarthria associated with cerebral palsy or other cerebral disease
3. Dysarthria associated with minimal signs of cerebral palsy
4. Isolated developmental dysarthria

Dyslalia
1. Transient defects of consonant omission and substitution

Stammering

movement of the soft palate; (3) dysarthria with clumsy movements of the tongue; and (4) dysarthria without apparent clumsiness of lips, tongue, or palate. In developmental dysarthria speech is slow and "clumsy" and may be punctuated by explosive words and phrases in severe cases. Imitation of speech is poor and omission errors dominate the pattern of speech production errors. These authors described general features of developmental dysarthria including an impressive history of speech defects in the family or a family tendency for speech problems; abnormal appearance and abnormal voluntary movements of the lip, tongue, or palate in a large number of the children; and associated disorders of language (including reading difficulty) in 50% (9 of 18 cases) of the children they studied, although the degree and characteristics of language impairment varied greatly. They stressed the importance of differentiating developmental dysarthria from dyslalia, which was described as a transient problem of consonant substitution in the absence of accompanying language impairment, and from "articulatory apraxia." One third (6 of 18 cases) of the children described in their 1954 paper demonstrated structurally normal lips, tongue, and palate; and the function of these structures appeared normal on voluntary movements carried out on request. However, movement of the same structures appeared clumsy and awkward when the children attempted "the more complex and rapid movements of articulation" (p. 9). This pattern was felt to reflect an articulatory apraxia.

Morley, Court, and Miller (1954) felt that the etiology of developmental dysarthria (including articulatory apraxia) was congenital and organic, specifically neurologic. They expressed the opinion that the underlying neurologic problem was focal cerebral dysgenesis similar to, but more limited than, that seen in congenital cerebral palsy, especially spastic diplegia.

In a related paper, Morley, Court, Miller, and Garside (1955) discussed developmental dysarthria and articulatory apraxia in reference to developmental aphasia. Aphasia was characterized as a language impairment containing a receptive component, an expressive component, or both. At this time these authors felt that, although developmental dysarthria might coexist with developmental aphasia, the two disorders bore no intrinsic relationship. The dysarthria could be readily identified by clinical examination and was not believed to "involve any interference with the internal comprehension and construction of words" (p. 463). Articulatory apraxia was, however, believed to share a special relationship with developmental aphasia—especially expressive. Their position was that these communicative disorders were related, possibly by proximity of neurologic "lesion," but that they were distinct clinical entities. They reported identification of several children presenting articulatory apraxia who demonstrated no evidence of language impairment. Likewise, they described children with aphasia (receptive and/or expressive) who demonstrated no evidence of articulatory apraxia. In specifying their impressions of the underlying neurologic etiology, they suggested that the "lesion" creating articulatory apraxia was at some point intermediate between that responsible for spastic dysarthria and the global failure of language development. Although Morley and her colleagues described dysarthria, apraxia, and aphasia as discrete disorders, they indirectly suggested a continuum of neurologically based communication problems: Developmental dysarthria at the purely motor end of the continuum, developmental aphasia at the purely language end of the continuum, and articulatory apraxia at some intermediate point. Figure 1–1 depicts the presumed relationships among these clinical entities.

Morley contributed significantly toward a better understanding of communicative problems in children. Her clinical descriptions and conceptualizations of these disorders were direct ancestors of much of the current thinking in this area worldwide, especially her views on articulatory apraxia in children. Another British clinical scientist, however, is responsible for some of the most significant insights into the disorder of isolated developmental dysarthria.

Developmental Dysarthria

Congenital Suprabulbar Paresis (Worster-Drought Syndrome)

A British physician and contemporary of Muriel Morley, C. Worster-Drought contributed significantly to understanding the disorder of developmental dysarthria. The disorder more commonly known as congenital suprabulbar pare-

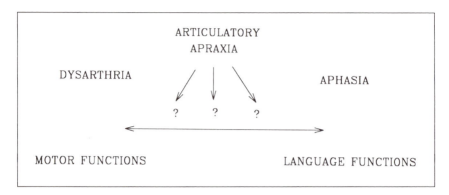

Figure 1–1. Continuum of neurologically based communication problems in consideration of the suggestions of Morley, Court, Miller, and Garside (1955).

sis also is referred to as Worster-Drought Syndrome. Worster-Drought (1953) suggested developmental dysarthria as an etiology for failure in speech development secondary to neurologic cause. This form of focal dysarthria in the absence of a more widespread cerebral palsy has not received significant attention outside of the writings of a few British authors. Worster-Drought published two summary papers that described the rationale for the label "congenital suprabulbar paresis" and the characteristics of children presenting this disorder (Worster-Drought, 1956, 1974). This condition has been presented under a variety of names including "pseudobulbar type of cerebral agenesis" and "pseudobulbar paralysis." According to Worster-Drought (1956):

> Congenital suprabulbar paresis does not appear to be very well known as a clinical entity. It consists of a more or less isolated weakness or paralysis of the muscular structures which derive their nerve supply through the medulla or bulb and thus includes the peripheral organs of speech. The paralysis dates from birth, is of the upper neurone type and varies in extent and degree in different cases. (p. 453)

Complete and Incomplete Versions of Congenital Suprabulbar Paresis

Worster-Drought (1956, 1974) described two general types of congenital suprabulbar paresis: complete and incomplete. As the name implies, the complete variety of the disorder represents the more severe form. In a 1974 monograph, 200 cases of congenital suprabulbar paresis seen over a 20-year period were reviewed. Forty-eight of the 200 cases (less than 25%) demonstrated the complete syndrome whereas 152 cases demonstrated the incomplete syndrome in varying degrees. A complete syndrome is characterized by a severe dysarthria with poor lingual and labial consonant production and a pronounced hypernasality in speech. Such children demonstrate inability to round the lips, severely restricted lingual mobility, and limited or no movement of the soft palate upon phonation or reflexive tasks. These children often demonstrate accompanying dysphagia or a history of swallowing difficulty. The dysphagia ranges in severity but may be sufficiently severe in some cases to preclude a normal oral diet. Vocal impairment (dysphonia), presumably related to weakness of the laryngeal muscles, may accompany the dysphagia.

Such children are expected to demonstrate abnormal reflexes within the facial musculature. Because the presumed etiology is in the supranuclear corticobulbar system, upper motor neuron reflexes such as a brisk jaw jerk and/or snout response may be present. Lower motor neuron signs, including atrophy or fasciculation, are not expected to be observed in the facial musculature. In most cases of the complete syndrome, the child has difficulty controlling his or her saliva. This is attributed to weakness within the lips and tongue and the associated impairment in swallowing. Children with the complete syndrome are often referred for uncontrollable drooling as well as for the severe and persistent speech problem.

The more common form of the disorder, the incomplete syndrome, was described as demonstrating a lesser degree of muscle weakness. The incomplete syndrome may be seen in various forms. Of the 152 cases who demonstrated the incomplete syndrome, the primary areas involved were: soft palate (68 cases), soft palate and tongue (34 cases), tongue and lip musculature (28 cases), and soft palate and lip musculature (22 cases). Figure 1–2 summarizes the distribution of anatomical involvement in the incomplete syndrome of congenital suprabulbar paresis. Worster-Drought suggested that it was not possible to further subdivide the incomplete syndrome into definite types because the extent and degree of paresis varies considerably.

Some degree of gradual spontaneous improvement may be expected as the children grow older, especially in the incomplete syndrome. This observation may be interpreted to represent a component of delayed neurological development versus deviant neurologic structure as an etiologic factor in this disorder. However, individuals with the complete syndrome have a much poorer expected outcome than those with the incomplete syndrome. Following the same line of reasoning, this observation may be interpreted to represent deviant neurologic structures as a causative factor, especially in severe cases of the complete syndrome. Table 1–2 compares salient characteristics of the complete versus incomplete variants of congenital suprabulbar paresis.

Congenital Suprabulbar Paresis: Concomitant Characteristics

In addition to the basic neuromotor, speech, and swallowing characteristics attributed to such children, Worster-Drought reported a variety of concomitant characteristics in children demonstrating congenital suprabulbar paresis. Included among these is some evidence of familial tendencies in this

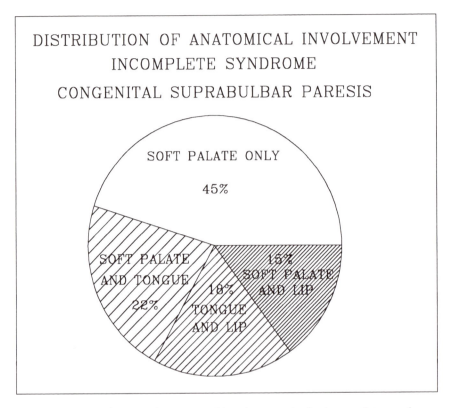

Figure 1-2. Distribution of anatomical involvement in the incomplete syndrome of congenital suprabulbar paresis. (Worster-Drought, 1974)

disorder. A wide range of intellectual ability was reported; however, the majority of children (58%) demonstrated average intelligence (IQ between 80–110). Seven percent of the children had performance IQs between 40 and 58. Worster-Drought noted that most of the children in the low range of intelligence demonstrated the complete syndrome of congenital suprabulbar paresis. He indicated that the prognosis for children with this problem depended greatly on their intelligence, possibly related to their ability to cooperate with various speech therapy techniques. One hundred and fifteen cases (57%) demonstrated additional congenital defects, in some cases multiple deficits in the same child. These included mild degrees of cleft palate in 7 cases (previously repaired), submucous clefts of the hard palate in 4 cases, tongue-tie (abnormally short lingual frenum) in 6 cases, "retarded development of spoken language other than defective articulation" in 62 cases (58 demonstrated predominantly expressive and four primarily receptive difficulties). Hearing impairment was found in 11 children, 5 with high frequency loss, 2 with low frequency loss, and 2 with deficits across all frequencies. Seven children suffered from epilepsy and 5 showed evidence of cerebellar

Table 1–2. Comparison of salient characteristics of the complete versus incomplete syndrome of congenital suprabulbar paresis according to Worster-Drought (1974).

Complete Syndrome (24%)	Incomplete Syndrome (76%)
Defective speech involving both lingual and labial consonants	Speech pattern dependent on selective involvement of lips, tongue, or velum
Hypernasality	Hypernasality only if soft palate involved
Limited lip and tongue movement	Paresis less severe than complete syndrome
Limited velar movement volitional or reflexive	Unlikely to find labial involvement
Dysphagia (or history of)	No dysphagia
Dysphonia	No dysphonia
Brisk jaw jerk reflex	Brisk jaw jerk reflex
Occasional snout reflex	
No atrophy	No atrophy
No fasciculation	No fasciculation
Possible intraoral sensory decrease	
Drooling	

dysfunction. Moebius Syndrome (agenesis of cranial nerve nuclei) was present in 6 children. Four of these demonstrated facial immobility and 2 demonstrated atrophy and fasciculation in the tongue. Four children had congenital heart defects, 3 had micrognathia and one child demonstrated Arnold-Chiari malformation. Three of the children with the incomplete syndrome were observed to "stammer." Most of the 200 cases he reports were slow in learning to read, and 14 of them were considered to have a specific developmental dyslexia. Table 1–3 summarizes the associated deficits of congenital suprabulbar paresis delineated by Worster-Drought (1974).

Worster-Drought on Treatment

In discussing management strategies for these children, Worster-Drought emphasized four major areas of concern: (a) dribbling (drooling), (b) immobility or weakness of the soft palate, (c) weakness of tongue movements, and (d) weakness of the lips. Worster-Drought favored surgical options in attempting to control drooling and improve velopharyngeal functions. He recommended speech therapy in mild cases of the incomplete syndrome, especially when surgery was not indicated. However, Worster-Drought (1974)

Table 1–3. Summary of congenital deficits concomitant with congenital suprabulbar paresis reported for 200 children by Worster-Drought (1974). Note that some of the deficits overlap in the same child. Therefore the total number of deficits exceeds the total number of children demonstrating concomitant deficits.

Deficit Area	Number of Children Demonstrating Deficit	
	Subgroup	Total
Language Difficulties		62
Primarily expressive	58	
Primarily receptive	4	
Dyslexia		14
Hearing Loss		11
High frequency only	5	
Low frequency only	2	
All frequencies	4	
Cleft Palate		7
Submucous only	4	
Epilepsy		7
Tongue Tie		6
Moebius Syndrome		6
Facial immobility	4	
Lingual atrophy and fasciculation	2	
Cerebellar Dysfunction		5
Congenital Heart Defects		4
Micrognathia		3
Stammering		3
Arnold Chiari Malformation		1
Total Number of Children Presenting Concomitant Deficits		115
Percent of Total Group (115/200)		57%

felt that "speech therapy is of little or no value for children with the complete syndrome, especially when the soft palate is completely paralysed" (p. 5). Speech therapy techniques were considered most useful in improving speech and swallowing functions after surgical intervention.

Congenital Versus Acquired Forms

It is important to note that Worster-Drought differentiated between congenital and acquired forms of suprabulbar paresis in children. Many causes of neurological dysfunction such as measles, encephalitis, traumatic injury, or other deficits may create an acquired suprabulbar paresis in children. In most cases, however, the neurological involvement extends beyond the cortico-bulbar system into the main pyramidal tract and elsewhere in the nervous system. In this regard there is often a degree of hemiparesis and possibly accompanying aphasia. The congenital form can be easily differentiated from the acquired form based on history. Worster-Drought also identified other aspects of the acquired form such as extrapyramidal rigidity in the facial muscles or facial paresis not limited to the lip musculature.

Case Examples of Congenital Suprabulbar Paresis

Following are two case histories adapted from Worster-Drought's 1974 monograph. The first case describes the incomplete syndrome. The second case describes the complete syndrome. The information in each has been summarized and edited; however, the author's original content is represented in each case.

Case 1

Description: Incomplete Syndrome involving orbicularis oris and tongue only: Normal speech attained with speech therapy.

J was seen at the age of nearly 8 years because of defective articulation. He is the older of two boys and the product of a normal and full-term pregnancy. He sat alone at 7 months and walked by himself at 16 months. By 2 years of age his parents realized he could not protrude his tongue, and they called their family doctor. Tongue-tie was ruled out and shortly afterwards the child was referred for speech therapy. J began to speak at 2½ years of age with isolated words which were difficult to understand from the onset. His parents understood him better than anyone else. His vocabulary gradually increased, and he did attend school at the age of 5 years. Initially, he had some difficulty learning to write and spell.

On examination, J was a rather nervous and excitable child. He was unable to round his lips or to grasp the mouthpiece of a toy trumpet. Other facial movements were normal. He could protrude his tongue only to just beyond his teeth, and he was unable to move the tongue from side to side or elevate it. There was no atrophy in the tongue musculature. His soft palate showed a full range of movement on phonation. He demonstrated a brisk and exaggerated jaw jerk. He was mildly dysphonic. Swallowing was apparently normal. There was no evidence of a hearing problem, and comprehension for spoken language was average for his age.

J had acquired a functional vocabulary, but his speech production was judged to be dysarthric. Analysis of speech patterns demonstrated primarily lingual and labial sounds in error. He was able to imitate all the vowels except "e," but many consonants were either not produced or were produced erroneously. He could not produce "g," "s," or "th." Words beginning with "l," "t," "d," and "n" were articulated by using the body of the tongue rather than the tip. He omitted "t," "k," "f," and "v" in the medial position and had difficulty with consonant blends. Sentence construction was good, although the sentences were brief. He was right-handed.

Intelligence testing, determined by two independent tests, indicated an IQ within the normal range. Vocabulary was estimated to be at the 8-year-old level, consistent with his age.

J was placed in a school for speech therapy and demonstrated good progress with his overall articulatory performance. [No specifics were provided regarding the speech therapy techniques nor the time spent in therapy.] Upon leaving the program, the lip musculature demonstrated mild weakness; however, he did manage to produce labial sounds quite well. Tongue movements had improved considerably. He could protrude the tongue almost fully and had lateral movement and even a slight upward curl. He did demonstrate a slight "slurring of lingual sounds," but otherwise adequate lingual articulatory skills. Palatal movement was normal, as it was on initiation of speech therapy, and fricative sounds were produced normally. At a 5-year follow-up, J's speech production gains had been well maintained; however he did continue to visit a local speech clinic once every 3 months for ongoing supervision.

Case 2

Description: Syndrome almost complete with severe drooling and hypernasality. Drooling was relieved by excision of the mandibular glands, and speech musculature showed gradual spontaneous improvement. This was the first case in which surgical treatment was attempted.

J was first seen at the age of 8 years. Since infancy he had noted difficulty in chewing and swallowing food and also in speech development. His speech was very slurred, hypernasal, and indistinct.

Birth history was uneventful. J had been bottle fed but demonstrated some difficulty in sucking and swallowing. He sat alone at 8 months, walked unsupported at 1 year, and began talking at 18 months. Speech production errors were evident from the onset of speech. He has a single brother with no relevant family history.

On examination, J could not round or purse his lips because of weakness in the orbicularis oris. Other facial muscles were within normal limits. J was able to elevate his tongue only slightly inside the mouth, but could not protrude it. Lateral movements were not possible. There was no atrophy of the tongue or fasciculation or tremor. The soft palate had only slight movement on phonation, and there was no palatal reflex. The palate and the pharynx appeared to have poor sensation. J did demonstrate difficulty in swallowing and was observed to push solid food to the back of his mouth using his finger. Drooling was considerable and the front of his clothes were often wet. He had normal jaw movement, but a hyperactive jaw jerk.

J's speech was considered to be extremely dysarthric with lingual and labial sounds being particularly deficient. He demonstrated considerable nasality in connected speech. He was unable to produce the "k" and "g" sounds in the initial position, and he produced defective sibilant sounds. He demonstrated no other abnormal neurologic signs. A barium swallow showed the pharynx and esophagus to be normally patent. Intelligence testing indicated an IQ of 100.

J was admitted to the school for speech therapy and received therapy for speech and swallowing on a regular basis. Following therapy some increase was noted in movement of the soft palate and of the tongue. One year after admission he could protrude his tongue slightly without support from the lower lip. Lateral movements were still not possible. Drooling was still pronounced at this time and was increased when tongue movements were attempted. Pharmacotherapeutic intervention produced only a slight and temporary reduction in the amount of drooling. Radiation therapy to the parotid glands was subsequently attempted; however, again there was only a slight and temporary reduction in the amount of drooling. One year later, surgical options were tried, but again the result was not satisfactory. A full year later, additional surgical options were attempted which resulted in considerable improvement in salivary control. At this time, J only drooled during periods of intense mental concentration, presumably because he forgot to swallow excess saliva. By the beginning of the following year, control of saliva had improved further. A final surgical technique was completed at this time and residual drooling was negligible. Over this period of time, there was an observed improvement in strength of the speech musculature and speech itself. Movement of the lip musculature, although far from normal, was adequate to produce labial sounds. Tongue protrusion increased; however, deficits were noted in lateral movement and tongue elevation, especially when attempted with protrusion. The soft palate was noted to have increased mobility, and there was no overt hypernasality in speech. Swallowing was nearly normal.

What's New Since Worster-Drought?

Aside from the extensive clinical descriptions offered by Worster-Drought through 1974 (this was, in fact, a posthumous publication coordinated by T. T. S. Ingram), very few references have focused specifically on congenital suprabulbar paresis. References have been scarce and scattered and typically have described the disorder only in reference to a related phenomenon.

Swallowing Difficulty

Weitz, Varsano, Geifman, Grunebaum, and Nitzan (1976) described a single infant with congenital suprabulbar paresis who demonstrated cricopharyngeal achalasia (basically, spasm in the muscle) as a component in a congenital swallowing problem. Severe dysphagia was present soon after birth and necessitated feedings via nasogastric tube. Over a 4-year period, there was evidence of spontaneous improvement in swallowing ability, and the child eventually was able to return to oral feeding. At age 4 years the child demonstrated "normal psychomotor development" and a good vocabulary, but defective articulation along with hypernasality, some difficulty with drooling, and persistent abnormal chewing and swallowing.

Evoked Potential Findings

Mason and Mellor (1984) studied auditory evoked potentials in children with speech or language disorders. Within the group of speech disordered children studied by these investigators were males with a motor speech disorder characterized as congenital suprabulbar paresis. These children demonstrated limited lingual protrusion, good lip spreading but poor lip pursing, and exaggerated jaw jerk, gag, and snout reflexes. They had difficulty with sucking, chewing, and swallowing, drooled, and were hypernasal with nasal air escape during speech. Auditory evoked potential findings suggested that children in this motor speech impaired group had an enhanced myogenic response much like other exaggerated brainstem reflexes seen in congenital suprabulbar paresis. These children also demonstrated larger cortical potentials at certain electrode sites. The authors attributed this to underactivity of normal cortical inhibitory systems. This study provides some objective support for a congenital deficit in the corticobulbar system in children demonstrating congenital suprabulbar paresis.

Familial Tendency

Patton, Baraitser, and Brett (1986) described familial tendencies of congenital suprabulbar paresis over three generations in a family. The focus of their study was a family originally seen by Worster-Drought in the 1950s. The disorder was observed in four males spanning three generations. Generations were spared such that unaffected males might have affected sons. The authors suggested that some cases of congenital suprabulbar paresis may be inherited as an autosomal dominant trait. One of their cases apparently developed normally until 2 years of age when he had an acute illness of unspecified origin which left him paralyzed below the waist. Recovery of motor functions in the legs was rapid (2 days); however, the child was reported to have stopped speaking, drooled excessively, swallowed poorly, and was unable to move his tongue. Further examination revealed evidence of the complete form of suprabulbar paresis. Based on this case, it was suggested that some individuals carry the gene for this syndrome and are predisposed to supranuclear damage in the corticobulbar system (especially cranial nerves 10 and 12), but the disorder is not expressed unless triggered by an environmental factor.

Pseudobulbar Palsy

Brown (1985) described what he refered to as pseudobulbar palsy in children. Although he did not use the term congenital suprabulbar paresis, he described the signs and behaviors that characterize the Worster-Drought syndrome. He mentioned Worster-Drought syndrome and described it as an unusual form of pseudobulbar palsy that presents in the neonatal period with feeding difficulties. It is characterized by delay in speech development and dysarthria with drooling, poor tongue and palatal movements, and a brisk jaw jerk. Feeding difficulties tend to disappear by 3 to 4 years of age. This occurs in isolation without any obvious spasticity in the muscles of the arms and legs. This disorder is differentiated from bulbar palsy and believed to be a developmental, probably genetically determined condition.

Some Points to Consider

Congenital suprabulbar paresis, or the Worster-Drought syndrome, is a well defined disorder of speech development. Yet, most of the clinical research describing this disorder to date was presented by two British authors nearly 40 years ago. More recent literature in speech-language pathology, specifically in the United States, has all but ignored this disorder of speech development. Perhaps the primary reason for the paucity of recent information on congenital suprabulbar paresis is the way speech-language problems have been approached in this country. Our tradition has been to focus on description rather than etiology and/or process. Given the range of difficulties presented by children with congenital suprabulbar paresis, they might be seen as cases of velopharyngeal insufficiency, severe phonological disorder, or even swallowing deficits. It is also likely that these children are grouped under the generic category of motor speech disorders without differentiation. However, given the potential benefit from the extensive descriptions offered by Worster-Drought, including differential prognoses, clinicians, and the children they treat, might have much to gain from a differential diagnostic perspective when trying to understand and manage children with suspected motor speech disorders. This perspective may lead us to more specific and effective clinical interventions.

If congenital suprabulbar paresis is erroneously grouped with other forms of developmental motor speech disorders, it is likely to be confused with its close relative—developmental apraxia of speech. The commonalities of the two disorders are deficits in motor speech performance. Differences across these conditions may be subtle. As an initial contrast between these disorders, the next section provides a brief historical perspective of developmental apraxia of speech.

Developmental Apraxia of Speech

A Rose by Any Other Name

Developmental apraxia of speech has been and remains a controversial entity in the field of communicative disorders. Part of the confusion and controversy surrounding this disorder is the result of dozens of names or labels applied to children who show unusual speech production patterns expected to be motoric in origin. Some of the names include articulatory apraxia, developmental apraxia of speech, developmental verbal apraxia, and, as seen in the prior section, developmental dysarthria or dysarthric apraxia. Another source of confusion is the variability of the characteristics attributed to children suspected to demonstrate this motor speech disorder. This point has been addressed by Guyette and Diedrich (1981) who do not support the clinical use of this label.

It is beyond the scope of this or any text at this juncture in history to argue definitively the case for utilizing this label to describe children with defective speech. Many unanswered questions cloud the argument. However, the reality that the concept of apraxia or dyspraxia has been applied to disorders of speech production in both adults and children cannot be ignored. In an attempt to understand the characteristics of developmental apraxia of speech (this term will be used as the primary descriptor throughout this text), a brief history of research and philosophy surrounding this concept may be beneficial.

Back to Morley

As previously stated, Morley and her colleagues first described articulatory apraxia as a subset of developmental dysarthria. Morley, Court, and Miller (1954) described a child with dysarthria in the absence of overt motor impairment to the lips, tongue, or palate. This child demonstrated severe speech impairment that persisted for several years despite intensive therapy efforts. The child had normal intelligence and no obvious structural-functional deficit in the oral articulators. The ability to imitate sounds in isolation or simple words was preserved; however, these productions were not incorporated in continuous speech. Subsequently, Morley, Court, Miller, and Garside (1955) used the term "articulatory apraxia" as a descriptor for a condition in which oral musculature appeared adequate for all functions other than highly complex movements of speech. This followed a tradition in neurology of referring to disturbances of movement that could not be attributed to weakness, paralysis, or involvement of specific muscle groups as "apraxias."

Given that the term "dysarthria" refers to a defect in articulation abilities, it is easy to understand Morley's position on the relationship between developmental dysarthria and articulatory apraxia. Developmental apraxia of speech is conceptually similar to the developmental dysarthria described by Morley and her colleagues. Essentially, this is a severe speech production disorder in the absence of overt signs of neuromuscular deficit within the oral mechanism, but with signs of motor dysfunction during speech production. Morley (1965) described this condition as follows:

> A defect of articulation which occurs when movements of the muscles used for speech (tongue, lips, palate) appear normal for involuntary and spontaneous movements such as smiling or licking the lips, or even for the voluntary imitation of movements carried out on request, but are inadequate for the complex and rapid movements used for articulation and the reproduction of the sequences of sounds used in speech. (p. 237)

Morley's contribution toward understanding development apraxia of speech is akin to that of Worster-Drought's clinical documentation of congenital suprabulbar paresis. In fact, although more recent investigators have discussed various attributes of developmental apraxia of speech, Morley's work still stands as one of the most comprehensive efforts in this area.

The Twelve Apraxics

Morley (1965) provided detailed longitudinal descriptions of 12 children she felt demonstrated developmental apraxia of speech. She followed the clinical progress of these 12 children (although one woman was 28 years at the time of referral) for time periods ranging from 1 to 7 years noting gender, intelligence, position in family, characteristics of speech development, family tendencies, emotional disturbance, oromotor dysfunction, pattern of speech errors, associated language disorders, prognosis, and persistence of the disorder.

Of the 12 individuals followed, 7 were boys and 5 were girls. These children had average or above average intelligence with performance scores ranging from 105 to 130. Two children were first born, six were born second, three were born third, and one born fourth. First words were observed between 10 months and 3 years of age with an average of 19 to 20 months. Phrases were noted on an average of 33 months with a range from 14 months to beyond 4 years. Family histories of speech disorder were obtained for 6 of the 12 children. Emotional disturbance was virtually absent in this group of children, although there was evidence of transient "anxiety" or emotional reactions to the speech disorder. None of the children demonstrated difficulty with volitional movement of the lips, tongue, or palate. During speech, however, oral movements were "awkward and misdirected." Speech production errors reflected a wide range of variability among the 12 children. There was an apparent range of severity from only a few consonant errors to most consonants omitted. Seven of the 12 children demonstrated severe articulation deficits, producing a limited number of consonants, whereas one child erred only a few consonants and another produced few errors in simple words but demonstrated increased errors as length of utterance increased. A few (number not specified) of the children demonstrated an associated language deficit (developmental aphasia) that persisted into the school years and beyond. Three children demonstrated a dyslexia, and one a persistent spelling disability. The outcomes for the 12 children studied by Morley appeared to be good. Six of the children demonstrated "normal" speech at or before 8 to 10 years of age, and only one girl was still considered unintelligible at 10 years of age. There were instances of persisting speech problems into adulthood. These tended to represent severe cases, and the persistent deficits covered a large range of severity. Table 1–4 presents a summary of the characteristics of the 12 children studied by Morley (1965).

It is obvious that there was a substantial degree of variability among the 12 children studied by Morley, especially in reference to speech and language abilities. The common denominator was the observed inability to perform accurate and coordinated oral movements during speech in the absence of oral movement deficits in nonspeech volitional motor tasks (no paresis). Morley seemed to attribute individual differences to severity. She did con-

Table 1–4. Summary of characteristics of 12 children with developmental apraxia of speech described by Morley (1965).

Gender	7 male and 5 female
Intelligence	Average or above average (Performance IQ = 105–130)
First Words	10 months–3 years (average 20 months)
Phrases	14 months–>4 years (average 33 months)
Family History	6/12 cases
Emotional Disturbance	Absent excepting transient "anxiety" in reaction to speech disorder
Paralysis/Paresis	None
Speech Pattern	Variable—yet, all children demonstrated "awkward and misdirected" oral movements during speech
Language Deficits	Variable—included deficits in both spoken and written language
Outcome	Good—"normal" speech attained in just over 50% of the children. Others demonstrated persistent deficits into adulthood

sider overlap between apraxia and dysarthria and/or aphasia, but she did not entertain the possibility of different forms of apraxia.

A Case in Point

Following is a case summary described by Morley (1965). It will be useful to contrast the salient features of this case with those of the congenital suprabulbar paresis cases presented previously.

F.S. was referred at 6 years. He was the fourth child and was born prematurely, weighing 3 pounds. His behavior during the first few weeks of life is not fully known, but at one stage "he was not expected to live." He did not dribble excessively, and there was no apparent difficulty in swallowing. He was walking at the age of 15 months and has always been a good runner. He did not begin to use words in any quantity until 2 years. When first seen he was a friendly and active boy with no abnormality in the nervous system apart from defective speech. This was fluent, but intelligible only to his parents. The tongue, lips, and palate were normal in appearance and movement, and he could sing accurately but still with defective articulation. Although at first progress was rapid and he was thought to have a simple dyslalia, the subsequent slowing down and failure to respond further to treatment suggested a more complex speech disorder. He had difficulty in imitating and using consonant sounds, and was helped considerably by watching the therapist's lips. When imitation of consonants was possible in isolation and in single words, he still had great difficulty in incorporating consonants correctly into speech. Two and a half years later articulation was still defective, and with increasing awareness of this, he became more cautious, often repeating words silently before speaking. He had difficulty in repeating phrases of a story and would change words, as in verbal paraphasia, or consonants, and often transpose them. . . . . At 9 years of age speech was usually intelligible. He also had some dyslexia, and at that time his reading age was only 6½ years. He had ceased to attend speech therapy but returned for help with reading, and at 10 years his reading age was 9 years. Articulation in spontaneous speech was then usually normal. His intelligence quotient on the Wechsler Bellevue Scale at 8 years was 113. On the verbal scale it was 108, and on the performance scale 121. (pp. 249–250)

Acquired Apraxia of Speech in Children

Morley (1965) describe acquired articulatory apraxia in children similarly to acquired suprabulbar paresis in children. She stated that in its developmental form acquired articulatory apraxia may occur in children with severe brain damage and a general motor disability. Furthermore, in such cases the apraxia may coexist with a dysarthria making a differential diagnosis difficult. Morley did not delineate specific differences between the congenital and acquired versions of developmental apraxia of speech as Worster-Drought did in the case of suprabulbar paresis. Rather, she provided a case example from which certain contrasting features may be inferred. In acquired cases there should be evidence of an event causing peri- or postnatal damage within the central nervous system. The child should show evidence of generalized motor deficit including the corticospinal system. This may take the form of a right hemiparesis. The child should not demonstrate a dysarthria. That is, the child should not demonstrate significant signs of corticobulbar deficit with related speech involvement. Finally, the child must demonstrate characteristics associated with apraxia of speech. As inferred from the work of Morley (1965), these characteristics include awkward/uncoordinated movement of the oral mechanism during speech, and articulation deficits. The basic behavioral characteristics of acquired apraxia of speech in children would seem to be the same as those of the congenital variety. The distinguishing feature between the two conditions appears to be the identification and reporting of an event in the medical history that specifically points to an onset of neurological damage.

What's New Since Morley

Since the extensive clinical documentations of Morley, there have been many papers describing aspects of developmental apraxia of speech or arguing for or against the conceptual and/or clinical bases of this disorder. However, few systematic, databased investigations have focused on this motor speech disorder. The 1960s and 1970s witnessed a significant increase in papers that focused on the possibility of a developmental apraxia of speech. Unfortunately, many of them contained little more than a rehashing of established ideas or opinions concerning this disorder. There were, however, some noteworthy additions to the body of literature in this arena.

Lingual Apraxia and Articulation Disorders

Palmer, Wurth, and Kincheloe (1964) evaluated a thousand consecutive cases of children with articulatory deficits. These children were given tests of lingual apraxia and agnosia (deficit in interpretation of sensory information). Of these 1,000 cases, 10.7% demonstrated lingual apraxia while an additional 2.4% demonstrated a combination of lingual agnosia and apraxia. Although Palmer and his colleagues were unable to specify lingual apraxia as a cause of these "functional articulation disorders," these authors reported that 8.6% of 70 cases of functional articulatory disorders demonstrated lingual apraxia. They concluded that, although the exact incidence of lingual apraxia is unknown, its presence does indicate a neurological component in so-called "functional articulatory disorders."

The Review: Rosenbek and Wertz (1972)

Rosenbek and Wertz (1972) reviewed 50 cases of developmental apraxia of speech in reference to neurological and speech and language findings. All of the children in their study demonstrated characteristics of developmental apraxia of speech, but some demonstrated other concomitant communication deficits (aphasia, 40%; dysarthria, 26%; or aphasia and dysarthria, 16%). The remaining children (18%) were believed to demonstrate an isolated apraxia of speech; however, the authors conceded that, due to limitations in language assessment and interpretation, concomitant language deficits in these cases may have been underestimated. Children with mental retardation were not excluded from their analysis.

Neurological Findings

Pediatric neurological evaluations were completed on 36 of the 50 children. The primary finding (22 of 36 cases) was generalized apraxia including oral apraxia (12 cases) or apraxia confined to orofacial musculature (7 cases). Fourteen of the 36 children demonstrated additional neurologic deficits including hyperreflexia and spasticity (8 cases), muscle weakness (3 cases), hyperkinesia (2 cases), and hyporeflexia and muscle weakness (1 case). Excessive drooling was present in 11 of the 50 children, 6 of whom demonstrated no paralysis or paresis in the oral mechanism. Difficulty in feeding during infancy was frequently reported (the authors did not indicate the exact frequency) for children with apraxia of speech both with and without dysarthria. Electroencephalographic (EEG) findings were reported for 26 of the 50 children. Eleven demonstrated normal EEGs, whereas 15 demonstrated either generalized or focal abnormalities. Ten of the children showed generalized cortical disturbances, two showed bilateral deficits (one in the motor strips, one in the temporoparietal areas), and three showed temporal and/or parietal disturbances in the right hemisphere only.

Speech Characteristics

Rosenbek and Wertz (1972) identified 13 speech and language characteristics in the 50 children demonstrating apraxia of speech. These are listed in Table 1–5. From these 13 traits, four characteristics were considered to be high probability indicators of an apraxic component. They were vowel errors, increasing number of errors in longer responses, a concomitant oral apraxia, and groping of the articulators.

The Rosenbek and Wertz (1972) report made two important contributions toward a better understanding of developmental apraxia of speech. This was one of the first studies to identify specific neurologic abnormalities within a group of children with apraxia of speech. This study also attempted to identify specific speech characteristics that might differentiate apraxia of speech from other articulatory disorders.

Table 1–5. Thirteen speech and language characteristics associated with developmental apraxia of speech according to Rosenbek and Wertz (1972).

1. May occur in isolation or in combination with aphasia and/or dysarthria.

2. Speech development is delayed and deviant.

3. Receptive abilities are inordinately superior to expressive abilities.

4. Oral nonverbal apraxia often, but not always, accompanies apraxia of speech.

5. Prominent phonemic errors: omissions (errors are more often omission of sounds and syllables than substitution of sounds and syllables), substitutions, distortions, additions, repetitions, prolongations.

6. Frequent metathetic errors.

7. Errors increase as words increase in length.

8. Repetition of sounds in isolation is often adequate; connected speech is more unintelligible than would be expected on the basis of single-word articulation test results.

9. Errors vary with the complexity of articulatory adjustment; most frequent errors are on fricatives, affricatives, and consonant clusters.

10. Misarticulations include vowels as well as consonants.

11. Errors are highly inconsistent.

12. Prosodic disturbances: slowed rate, even stress, and even spacing perhaps in compensation for the problem.

13. Groping trial-and-error behavior manifested as sound prolongations, repetitions, or silent posturing which may precede or interrupt imitative utterances.

Controlled Comparisons: Yoss and Darley (1974a)

Perhaps the best known experimental study of developmental apraxia of speech was completed by Yoss and Darley (1974a). These investigators compared a group of children with speech disorder to a group of children with normal speech, and subsequently divided the speech disordered group into two subsets. They compared their subjects on the basis of speech diadochokinetic performance, speech articulation performance, nonspeech tests of oral praxis, auditory perception and discrimination, and neurological examination results. Yoss and Darley concluded that there was evidence to support the concept of developmental apraxia of speech as a subset of children with articulation disorders. They divided their group of children with defective articulation into two subgroups based on performance on a task of isolated volitional oral movements (i.e., puff out your cheeks, show me how you blow, etc.). Significant intergroup differences were found on tasks of sequential oral movement (sequences of the individual movements), neurologic ratings (primarily motor indices), and certain speech production tasks (sequencing the syllable "kuh," voicing errors, and maintaining syllabic integrity within polysyllabic words).

They reported no significant group differences on any of the auditory perception or discrimination tasks. In attempting to identify characteristics that might differentiate developmental apraxia of speech from other articulatory disorders, Yoss and Darley completed a discriminant function analysis using 13 speech error variables and the neurologic rating for each child. The neurologic rating emerged as the strongest "discriminator" between the two subgroups of children with defective articulation along with seven types of speech errors: two and three feature errors, prolongations and repetitions, additions, distortions, one-place errors, and omissions.

The Yoss and Darley (1974a) investigation remains one of the few attempts to experimentally validate the concept of developmental apraxia of speech. Their results suggested that such children demonstrate more neurologic deviations and different speech production characteristics than either normal speaking children or other children with articulatory disorders.

A Challenge to Yoss and Darley

The Yoss and Darley (1974a) study received a strong challenge from Williams, Ingham, and Rosenthal (1981). These investigators attempted to replicate the Yoss and Darley study and found only partial support for the earlier results. A primary disagreement between the two studies was the paucity of neurologic soft signs observed among the children with articulation disorders in the Williams et al. study. Also, although they replicated some of the Yoss and Darley findings (i.e., speech diadochokinetic performances), there were truly more differences than similarities between the results of the two studies. These differences lead Williams and her colleagues (1981) to conclude that "none of the data in this study could be interpreted as identifying a developmental apraxia of speech" (p. 502). This conclusion reflects the argumentative tone of discussions that have encumbered the concept of developmental apraxia of speech for many years. Two important observations from the Williams et al. study must be considered in light of their conclusion.

Despite intensive efforts to complete a detailed replication of the Yoss and Darley (1974a) study, there were procedural differences in the Williams et al. investigation. Specifically, there were differences in the speech articulation abilities of the control groups between the two studies. Control subjects in the replication study demonstrated greater variability and poorer articulatory performances than those in the Yoss and Darley study. Since key comparisons in each study were dependent on the performance of the control group, this difference may have had a critical influence on the resulting discrepancies between the two studies.

A second, perhaps more important consideration of the replication study is that of perspective. One has to wonder if these investigators have missed the forest while counting the trees. Procedural differences aside, Williams, Ingham, and Rosenthal (1981) did find differences both between the control and articulation disordered groups and between subsets of the articulation disordered group. Some of these differences were the same as those reported by Yoss and Darley (1974a) while others were not, but there were differences. Perhaps, as stated by Williams and her colleagues (1981), "the two studies simply may have described two different groups of children with articulation disorders" (p. 504). Or, perhaps the finding that the exact nature of the observed differences deviated between the two studies reflects variability within a subset of children with apparent motor speech limitations. This speculation raises the possibility that there may be more than a single unvarying subset of children with motor speech disorders. The contrasts between these two important studies also raise into question the way in which any disorder is defined.

A Different Perspective: Aram's Contributions

Beginning in 1979, Dorothy Aram presented and/or published a series of papers that evaluated various aspects of what she referred to as developmental verbal apraxia. Aram's (Aram & Nation, 1982) position was that multiple components of the expressive grammar were involved in the disorder and she advocated the term developmental verbal apraxia versus developmental apraxia of speech to include the linguistic aspects of the disorder, emphasizing that "articulatory and language disorders do not simply coexist, but that both stem from a common breakdown in the selection and sequencing of both language and articulatory elements" (p. 165). In a rather extensive study of 8 children, Aram and Glasson (1979) evaluated phonologic, phonetic, language, and neurologic characteristics believed to be associated with developmental verbal apraxia. Based on the findings of that study and considering previous findings of various investigators, Aram offered 10 characteristics attributed to children demonstrating developmental verbal apraxia. These are summarized in Table 1–6.

In addition to detailing speech characteristics, Aram and Glasson (1979) completed detailed evaluations of language abilities in their eight subjects. Their results led them to consider that developmental verbal apraxia was as much a language-based disorder as an articulation-based disorder. This perspective extended the earlier views of Morley, Rosenbek and Wertz, and others who focused on overlapping but separate deficits in speech versus language ability. Aram's position focused on a common underlying process for both speech and language disturbances. Finally, in evaluating neurologic findings in their subjects, Aram and Glasson found little evidence supporting a focal cortical disturbance. Aside from a variety of associated gait and coordination problems, only two of their subjects demonstrated any neurologic irregularities. Both of these showed posterior hemisphere deviations on computerized tomography (CT) scans. These findings contrast somewhat with the relatively high incidence of neurologic abnormalities reported by Rosenbek

Table 1-6. Aram's "criteria for developmental verbal apraxia revisited."

1. Children demonstrate a contrast in their voluntary versus nonvoluntary use of the speech articulators.

2. Their disorder is notably one of selection and sequencing of both phonologic and articulatory movements, typically exemplified in difficulties in repetition of multisyllabic words or "puh-tuh-kuh."

3. They have essentially normal (if mental age is normal) language comprehension abilities but disordered lexical and syntactic formulation.

4. They present learning difficulties in some instances, particularly in reading, written expression, and spelling.

5. Their condition improves slowly and is often highly resistant to therapy used for other articulatory disorders.

6. They present some positive neurologic findings, including difficulties with fine and gross motor coordination, although neurologic findings are usually nonfocal.

7. They usually, but not always, have an accompanying oral apraxia of nonspeech movements.

8. They often fail to show a clear hand preference.

9. They typically are boys.

10. They often have a strong family history of speech, language, and learning problems.

Source: Adapted from Aram, D., & Nation, J. (1982). *Child language disorders* (pp. 165–166). St. Louis: C. V. Mosby.

and Wertz (1972); however, both studies failed to identify any focal cortical deficits based on neurologic examination, electroencephalography (EEG), or CT findings.

Back to the Future: Crary's Perspective

Crary (1984a) approached developmental apraxia of speech as a motor speech disorder resulting from congenital deficits in cortical mechanisms responsible for various components of speech control. This perspective seemed closer to traditional thinking than to Aram's position, but there were important distinctions from the more traditional motor speech orientation. Working from descriptions of the apraxias as a group of motor disorders rather than a unitary disorder, Crary developed the hypothesis that there was possibly more than one form of developmental apraxia of speech. By comparing neurologic functions associated with both speech-language and motor performance, he postulated that developmental apraxias of speech were "motolinguistic" disorders of speech-language development in which speech and motor characteristics would demonstrate parallel deficits. This position will form the basis for much of the approach to developmental motor speech disorders found in this book and is developed further in Chapters 2 and 3.

Implications and Considerations

Clinicians have long recognized differences among children with disorders of speech production. Certain children present with obvious neuromuscular deficits in the oral musculature. Some of these children are best described as presenting a form of dysarthria termed congenital suprabulbar paresis or Worster-Drought syndrome. An additional group of children appear to demonstrate severe motoric deficits during speech production in the absence of focal neuromotor signs. Initially considered to present a "developmental dysarthria," the characteristics demonstrated by these children have gradually become associated with the concept of apraxia. Subsequently, these children have been described by the term developmental apraxia of speech. A third group of speech-disordered children exists that has been referred to historically as demonstrating dyslalia, characterized by transient and relatively mild speech articulation deficits. Finally, a group of communicatively impaired children has been described who present more encompassing language disorders with both receptive and expressive deficits. The presence of a more generic language dysfunction in the child does not preclude the presence or coexistence of a dysarthria or an apraxia of speech.

Much confusion and controversy continues to surround the "not-so-obvious" motor speech disorders seen in certain children. Most clinicians can agree on the presence of some degree of motor dysfunction in these children, yet questions remain about the exact nature of the observed motor deficits, the relationship of these deficits to the speech disorder, the role of expressive language deficits, and other basic clinical questions. To address some of these questions, the remaining chapters of this book will be based on the formulation of a neurologic model that attempts to incorporate and account for these variants of developmental speech disorders and evaluate their relationships to each other. Subsequent chapters will delineate clinical profiles of individuals with these disorders including motor and motor speech performance, speech production and language abilities, and potential relationships to other developmental learning disabilities. All of this formulation, interpretation, description, and delineation provides the infrastructure and foundation for the primary objective of this book: Attempting to outline strategies for assessment and management of these children that will instill a more acceptable quality to their communicative lives.

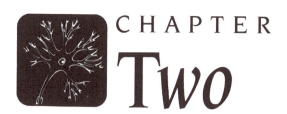

CHAPTER

Two

Theoretical Underpinnings: A Neurolinguistic Perspective

Why does any child have difficulty learning to speak? Why do some children "outgrow" speech difficulties while others demonstrate persistent deficits into adulthood? Historically, many possibilities have been considered, including environmental, genetic, and neurologic factors. Consider for a moment that these are not isolated causative agents, but rather form a potential triad of precipitating factors that might result in poor speech production. Within the framework of motor speech disorders it is tempting to look for cause among neurologic factors. Even in the absence of "hard" neurologic findings such as obvious paralysis and/or sensory deficits, many children with speech disorders demonstrate signs of neurologic dysfunction. Many of these signs "disappear" as the child develops, and in many cases, the speech production deficit changes or disappears as well. This chapter examines potential contributing factors to speech disorders in children and offers a neurolinguistic perspective from which to conceptualize these disorders.

Implied Neurologic Bases of Developmental Motor Speech Disorders

The implications for neurological dysfunction in developmental motor speech disorders are obvious. Worster-Drought (1974) described a dysarthria of the upper motor neuron variety with abnormal reflexes in postulating a "lesion" in the corticobulbar tract as the cause of congenital suprabulbar paresis. Morley and colleagues (1955) hypothesized that the "lesion" responsible for developmental apraxia of speech is somewhere between the "lesion" contributing to dysarthria and that contributing to developmental aphasia. These authors use the term "lesion" in somewhat of a theoretical application. The disorders emphasized by Worster-Drought and Morley are congenital. They do have acquired counterparts resulting from post-natal injury to the central nervous system, but these have different clinical characteristics (see Chapter 1). As demonstrated in the work of Rosenbek and Wertz (1972) and Aram and Glasson (1979), few of the children with the congenital form of these disorders demonstrate measurable signs of "hard" neurological dysfunction. Yet, despite variations in the specifics of the overt speech disorder, many of these children present a cluster of characteristics that may point to an underlying, congenital dysfunction in the central nervous system. The basic pattern includes: Concomitant speech and nonspeech motor deficits; frequent overlap with language, especially expressive language, deficits; tendency for familial predisposition; and high incidence of related learning disabilities—especially difficulty with reading. An additional commonality that cannot be ignored is the tendency for many of these children to "outgrow" these disorders. That is, the severity, if not the presence, of developmental motor speech disorders tends to diminish with age and development. These clinical observations point to two questions, the answers to which may provide a better understanding of developmental motor speech disorders:

1. Is there evidence of abnormal neurological development among children with motor speech disorders? If so, what is the potential nature of the neurological dysfunction? and

2. What are the relationships among motor, speech, language, and other learning deficits in children with developmental motor speech disorders?

To address these questions, this chapter will present a review of normal central nervous system development with implications for development of speech and language functions, describe sources of potential disruption in neurologic development that might contribute to behavioral developmental deficits, and consider mechanisms that may account for observed overlap among motor, speech, language, and related functions.

From Synapse to System: A Brief Overview of Central Nervous System Development

Traditional Models: Step by Step Development

There are at least two perspectives regarding maturation of human cortex and the development of functional systems. Traditionally, a hierarchical model of cortical development has been proposed. On the basis of indices such as brain weight, dendritic proliferation, and myelination (Altman, 1967; Conel, 1939–1963; Flechsig, 1901; Yakolev & Lecours, 1967), this model has proposed that the primary sensory and motor projection areas are the first to mature, followed in sequence by secondary (projection-association) areas, and finally by tertiary (association-association) areas.

A typical example of neurological maturation from this perspective is the degree of dendritic proliferation noted in various anatomic subsystems. Poliakov (1961) and DeCrinis (cited by Lenneberg, 1967) separately reported different patterns of dendritic growth for different cortical areas. The first areas to reach dendrogenic maturity are the primary projection areas of vision and audition and the pre- and post-Rolandic strips for sensory and motor functions. The next areas to mature are the secondary association areas that receive input from the projection areas. These areas mature at approximately 2 years of age. The final stage of maturation begins between the ages of 2 and 4 years. During this time period, parts of the frontal and parietal lobes (tertiary association areas) begin to mature. Thus, primary sensory and motor areas develop first, followed by their modality-related association areas (secondary fields). Regions of inter-area association (tertiary fields) are the last to develop.

A Different View of Development: Pruning Back the Overgrowth

Recent studies of brain growth in both primates and humans have provided an alternative model for describing cortical development. Rakic, Bourgeois, Eckenhoff, Zecevic, and Goldman-Rakic (1986) examined pre- and postnatal synaptogenesis in five areas of macaque cerebral cortex. They expected to identify differential growth patterns supporting a hierarchical model, but they instead identified more homogenous synaptogenesis in all areas and layers of cortex examined. In other words, neuronal connections seemed to proliferate at about the same time in all areas of the cortex. During the last 2 months of gestation, synaptic density increased at a rapid rate in all cortical areas examined, reaching a level equivalent to that of the sexually mature adult macaque. Synaptic density increased to levels much higher than that of the adult during the first 4 postnatal months. Subsequently, a reduction of synapses was noted that was rapid at first and then more gradual. This study suggests that the macaque brain develops as a whole rather than hierarchically and implies that functional subsystems may be an outgrowth of synaptic "pruning" postnatally. Huttenlocher (1979) has demonstrated a similar pattern of synaptic overproduction in the human cortex. The implication of these observations is that, both in the human child and the nonhuman primate, functional neuromaturation may result from synapse elimination facilitating the development of subsystems to mediate more refined behaviors.

Neurological Models and Speech and Language Development

Jason Brown (1979) has suggested a similar model of neurological maturation in explanation of language functions and disorders. He reviewed findings concerning neurological maturation in both human and nonhuman species that "are in agreement with concept of an evolutionary and maturational progression from a diffuse to a focal organization . . ." (p. 143). He contends that focal cortical areas develop out of generalized neocortex. This phylogenetic approach proposed by Brown appears to share points of agreement with the more recent findings of Rakic et al. (1986). The resulting model appears to be the converse of the more traditional hierarchical model. However, both views recognize the developmental importance of cortical functional subsystems. In this respect, the two views have similar implications for speech-language development. Both would predict that early behaviors would reflect more diffuse/nonfocal processes and that development of more refined/analytic behaviors would result from maturation of specific subsystems. Thus, although there are questions concerning the precise nature of neurological maturation relevant to speech-language development, the functional interpretations may be similar at various behavioral levels.

Hemispheric Development: Implications for Speech-Language Functions

Growth in the Respective Hemispheres: Lead with Your Right

Spoken language functions rest primarily within the domain of the left hemisphere. This concept is generally accepted as a neurolinguistic truism. A presumed neurologic basis for this "dominance" pattern is the asymmetry in size of language areas between the hemispheres. Geschwind and Levitsky (1968), in postmortem studies, reported that language areas of the left hemisphere (planum temporale and perisylvian areas) were larger than corresponding areas of the right hemisphere. This observation has been repeatedly documented using a variety of techniques in adult brains (Falzi, Perrone, & Vignolo, 1982;

Wada, Clarke, & Hamm, 1975), in neonates (Witelson & Pallie, 1973), and in prenatal brains (Chi, Dooling, & Gilles, 1977). This asymmetry is presumed as a biological basis for speech-language dominance within the left hemisphere. However, although it is true that, in adults, left hemisphere damage impairs speech-language functions more often than right hemisphere damage, the right hemisphere also has identifiable language ability (Zaidel, 1985). And, from a developmental perspective, the right hemisphere may demonstrate a maturational lead over the left hemisphere in areas thought to govern speech-language functions. Simonds and Schiebel (1989) studied dendritic growth in right and left hemisphere frontal lobe areas believed to be associated with oral movement (inferior portion of primary motor strip) and motor speech control (Broca's area) in infant brains between 3 and 72 months of age. Their results indicated an early "dominance" of right hemisphere dendritic systems with a gradual shift to left hemisphere dominance. These investigators also observed more advanced development in oral motor areas over motor speech areas in younger specimens, but a reversal of this pattern with development. The timing of these patterns of neuromaturation was such that up to approximately 12 months the right hemisphere showed more advanced development than the left. From 1 year to between 2 and 4 years the left hemisphere "catches up," and by approximately 4 years of age the left hemisphere showed more advanced neuronal development on many, but not all, indices of maturation. A similar timetable was observed for development of oral motor versus motor speech areas. In the youngest specimens the oral motor areas showed advanced development over the motor speech areas. Between 2 and 3 years of age the motor speech areas surpassed the primary oral motor areas in neuronal complexity and maintained this neurologic advantage.

There seems to be a built-in left hemisphere potential for speech-language functions. However, this potential must be realized through processes of neuromaturation (and variables that influence these processes). The progression of neuromaturation might be expected to correspond to observed behavioral changes in speech-language functions. Crary, Voeller, and Haak (1988) offered a preliminary model of developmental neurolinguistic functions that attempted to depict this presumed relationship (Table 2–1). These authors suggested similar patterns of neuromaturation (specifically hemispheric relations) and related them to changes in speech-language development. Crary, Voeller, and Haak (1988) hypothesized that certain speech-language deficits may reflect incomplete or deviant maturation of various "neurolinguistic subsystems." Furthermore, they suggested that children demonstrating certain speech-language disorders may be "stuck" between stages of language development as a result of deviant neuromaturation. One implication of this hypothesis is that the expected shift from right to left dominance is incomplete or deviant and that resultant left hemisphere subsystems subsequently failed to develop in the expected manner. To aid evaluation of this possibility, a re-

Table 2–1. Preliminary model of developmental neurolinguistic functions offered by Crary, Voeller, and Haak (1988).

Age Range	Anatomic Subsystem	Hemispheric Relations	Language Stage	Language Mode	Representative Skills
0–8 mos.	Primary projection (sensory and motor)	Primarily subcortical control and/or diffuse cortical systems	Prelinguistic	Reflexive (preintent)	1. S → R crying and cooing 2. Voice and face recognition 3. Prosodic recognition and imitation
8–12 mos.	Primary projection Growth in corpus callosum Growth in projection association system	Right > Left	Prelinguistic	Intent	1. Increased intentional communication (pragmatics) 2. Onset of first words
1–2 yrs.	Projection–Association	Right > Left or Right = Left	Lexical	Semantic (gestalt)	1. Increased vocabulary 2. Preliminary phonological development 3. Initial word combinations
2–4 yrs.	Association–Association	Left > Right	Grammatic	Sequential/ Analytic	1. Phonological growth 2. Syntactic growth 3. Continued growth in all language areas

Source: From Crary, M. A., Voeller, K., & Haak, N. J. (1988). Questions of developmental neurolinguistic assessment. In M. Tramontana & S. Hooper (Eds.), *Assessment issues in child neuropsychology* (p. 271). New York: Plenum Press.

view of speech-language functions attributed to the right and left hemispheres is presented.

Right Hemisphere Contributions

Zaidel (1979, 1985) contended that the right hemisphere is capable of performing a variety of linguistic tasks comparable to that of language-normal children between 3 and 6 years of age. A right-hemisphere language strength is a degree of auditory comprehension. However, this is adversely affected by length of input (limited short-term verbal memory) and grammatical structure/content. The right hemisphere seems to be most adept at language tasks involving semantic interpretation. The right hemisphere is believed to have very limited phonological abilities, but can comprehend auditory input by taking a direct path from acoustic information to semantic analysis. This trait also influences reading ability. The right hemisphere has little or no grapheme-phoneme conversion abilities, that is, the skills necessary to transfer between written and spoken language functions.

Speech characteristics of the right hemisphere depend on the technique used to study the question. For most people, speech is a left-hemisphere phenomenon. There are individuals, however, with "right-hemisphere speech." Examples of this include cases of crossed-aphasia in which a right-hemisphere lesion precedes aphasic impairment (Albert, Goodglass, Helm, Rubens, & Alexander, 1981). In addition, studies using the sodium amytal procedure (WADA test) to anesthetize one hemisphere at a time have reported observations of speech located within the right hemisphere (Ratcliff, Dila, Taylor, & Milner, 1980). Wada, Clarke, and Hamm (1975) reported that, when the speech dominant hemisphere (left) is inactivated, many patients retain the ability to produce automatic speech and melodic expression. Thus, it seems that the right hemisphere has some speech capacity and may be dominant for speech in certain individuals.

Studies with hemispherectomized children also implicate the reality of right-hemisphere speech. Dennis and Whitaker (1976) reported the results of language testing on two children who had the left hemisphere removed prior to speech development. Both of these children were observed to develop comparable manual and verbal expression abilities. At 9 years of age these children were assessed to be functioning approximately 2 to 3 years below age expectations on tests of manual and verbal expression. These developed functions were, however, among the poorest language abilities for these children. The same pattern did not result in a child following right hemisphere removal. Apparently, even in such drastic cases as left-hemispherectomy, there is evidence that the right hemisphere has some expressive capacity (manual and verbal) although it is inferior to the left hemisphere's capacity for these functions.

Zaidel (1985) summarized right hemisphere speech-language functions as follows:

This profile is characterized by better language comprehension than expression and better auditory comprehension than reading. Reading proceeds "ideographically," without intermediate phonological representation. The profile includes a rich lexical semantic organization and supports some conventional aspects of nonverbal communication, but has limited syntax and phonology. Cognitively, it is characterized by a limited STVM (short term verbal memory). This profile does not correspond to any stage in natural language acquisition. (p. 225)

Right, Left, or Both Hemispheres?

Zaidel (1985) believed that both hemispheres may participate interactively in speech-language development up to 3 to 6 years of age. Following this period, right-hemisphere aspects that are less efficient than those in the left hemisphere (i.e., speech) are functionally suppressed. Other characteristics that are effectively modulated by the right hemisphere (i.e., lexical comprehension) remain there. He believes that different components of speech-language "lateralize to or specialize in" the left hemisphere to varying degrees and have different neurological histories (p. 215). Crary, Voeller, and Haak (1988), in consideration of Zaidel's contention, have suggested that the asymmetrical shift of certain language functions "may be a phenomenon of the demands of a maturing linguistic system in cooperation with specific neurological growth or change" (p. 258). In short, the left hemisphere may be designed better to facilitate certain speech-language functions. Curtis (1985) has taken this position even further, suggesting that development of "computational" aspects (herein implicating structural, grammatical aspects of spoken language) may be a trigger for cerebral lateralization of many functions. She postulates that if language acquisition is disrupted other lateralized asymmetries may not develop.

This position raises interesting questions in the event of abnormal neurologic development within the left hemisphere. If the left hemisphere is designed to accept and house certain language functions, and if the left hemisphere is impaired in its ability to accept these functions by maturational irregularities, it is possible that either the right hemisphere will continue to mediate these functions, albeit inefficiently, or the left hemisphere must develop alternate systems (subsystems) to mediate these functions. In either case, one would expect a disruption in the normal timetable of speech-language acquisition related to left-hemisphere processes. Subsequent speech-language abilities would either reflect the more "gestalt" processes of the right hemisphere and/or deficient "analytic" processes of the left hemisphere. The implications are that children with deficient speech-language abilities would demonstrate change in performance with continued development; however, they would be expected to show continued limitations in various linguistic processes associated with left-hemisphere functions.

Left Hemisphere Contributions: Neurolinguistic Subsystems

In adults, lesions to different areas of the left hemisphere are known to result in differential impairment to speech-language abilities. This clinical observation has led many investigators to postulate the existence of "centers" of function associated with various skills (e.g., Hecaen & Albert, 1978).

Kent and McNeil (1987), building on observations of Darley, Aronson, and Brown (1975) and Mlcoch and Noll (1980) offered the conceptual model of speech processing depicted in Figure 2–1. This model, offered to help explain apraxia of speech in adults, should not be regarded as "anatomically correct." The general locations of various functions are loosely accepted, but studies attempting to relate specific brain areas to speech functions in adult apraxic speakers have not supported a high degree of localization specificity (Marquardt & Sussman, 1984). Because this model focuses on motor speech processes, a closer look is warranted.

The auditory speech processor (ASP) functions as a phonetic analyzer. Output from the ASP is considered a phonetic representation of the intended utterance. At this point, analyzed auditory information is believed to contain little meaning. ASP output is directed either to the central language processor (CLP) or to the articulatory coder (AC). The CLP is responsible for se-

Figure 2–1. Conceptual model of left-hemisphere speech processes from Kent and McNeil (1987, p. 193, with permission).

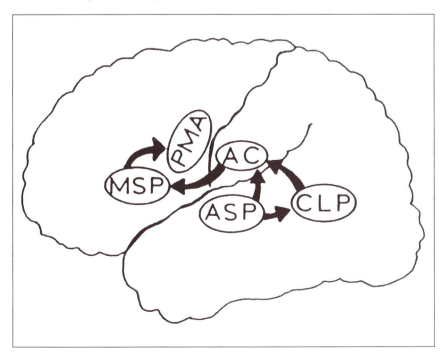

mantic interpretation. It also is thought to transform semantically interpreted information to prepare it for use by motor areas. This may be the general area where lexical items (words) are selected and phonologically organized (e.g, Cappa, Cavalotti, & Vignolo, 1981). This information is forwarded to the AC which is thought to convert phonetic (information arriving from the ASP) or possibly phonologic (information arriving from the CLP) information into articulatory specifications. This area (the AC) seems to be the architect of motor speech programming. Here, plans or blueprints for speech are developed. The information guiding these plans may be semantically potent, arriving from the CLP, or semantically void, arriving from the ASP. The articulatory plans generated by the AC are forwarded to the motor speech programmer (MSP). The MSP converts the articulatory code into motor programs. These programs (possibly a complex set of neuromotor instructions) are enacted via the primary motor area (PMA).

These anatomic and functional perspectives offered in Kent and McNeil's model raise an interesting question: "Is there more than one way to produce speech?" One answer to this question is found in a study of three adults with aphasia completed by McCarthy and Warrington (1984). In consideration of speech production errors in spontaneous speech versus repetition in two conduction and one transcortical motor aphasic patients, these investigators suggested a two-route model of speech production (Figure 2–2).

The crux of this model is the area or level of processing termed "semantic/phonological transcoding." This aspect of speech processing is impaired in the person with transcortical motor aphasia resulting in phonological deficits in spontaneous speech (a condition in which semantic processing is deemed a necessary input to phonological coding) with spared phonological coding in repetition tasks (presumably a more automatic task not requiring semantic interpretation). Conversely, individuals with conduction aphasia demonstrated deficits in the other "route," sparing semantic input to the phonological system but impairing the more automatic link between auditory input and articulatory output. McCarthy and Warrington believed that this pattern of performance reflected a deficit in phonological processing, whereas the performance pattern in the transcortical motor patient reflected an impairment between semantic analysis and speech production. An interesting result from this study was that individuals with spared semantic functions (conduction aphasia) demonstrated improved speech production in tasks that maximized active semantic processing. The converse result was obtained from the individual with transcortical aphasia.

The results of the McCarthy and Warrington (1984) study imply two active routes for speech production that are functionally different. Furthermore, when one route is impaired, function may be facilitated by manipulating aspects of speech production related to other processing levels within that system. It is conceivable, therefore, that children demonstrating severe speech production disorders early in life may show improved speech production by

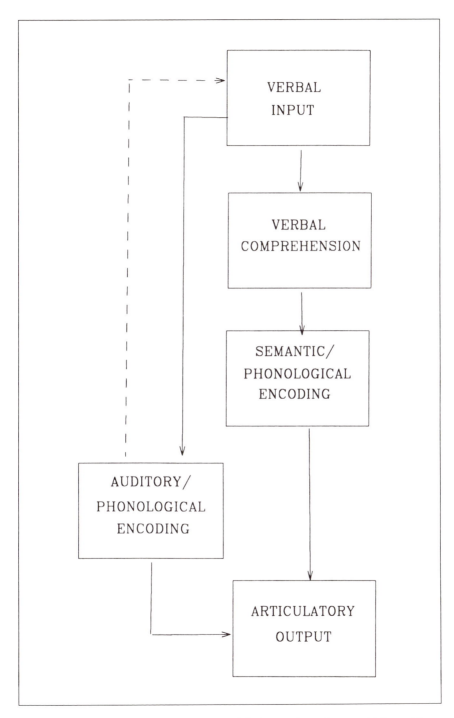

Figure 2–2. Schematic of a two-route model of speech production. (Adapted from McCarthy & Warrington, 1984)

using an alternative route or by enhancing function in a related level of speech processing within the same route.

Implications for Speech-Language Disorders in Children

Adults Versus Children

Because the models just described were developed from studying acquired speech-language deficits in adults, it is fair to question their application to children with disorders of speech-language performance. A cavalier response might be to point out that children grow into adults, and therefore speech-language development reflects growth of these various left-hemisphere neurolinguistic subsystems. Unfortunately, this position does not account for the potential flexibility of neurolinguistic development. We know, for example, that removal of the left hemisphere in a young child does not preclude some degree of speech-language development. The same procedure might prove linguistically disastrous in an adult. Also, children who suffer post-natal neurological deficits leading to acquired aphasia do not demonstrate aphasic "syndromes" similar to their adult counterparts. Reports of childhood aphasia typically depict initial muteness followed by nonfluent, telegraphic speech with relatively spared comprehension. There are few reports of posterior left-hemisphere language symptoms such as paraphasias, fluent speech, and reduced auditory comprehension (Satz & Bullard-Bates, 1981). If auditory comprehension is impaired, it is typically a transient impairment (Hecaen, 1976) or present in older children (VanDongen, Loonen, & VanDongen, 1985). Such patterns of linguistic impairment in childhood-acquired aphasia are not exceedingly helpful in proposing left-hemisphere neurolinguistic subsystems from a developmental perspective.

Developmental Speech-Language Disorders

There is, however, a separate, larger group of children with speech-language impairments who do present different profiles of deficits at an early age—and they demonstrate change over time. Examination of subtypes of developmental speech-language disorders may support the concept of developing neurolinguistic subsystems. Reports by Aram and Nation (1975) and Denckla (1981) using different techniques of study have suggested the presence of global speech-language deficits as well as more selective deficits involving naming, repetition, speech production, and/or comprehension impairments. Rapin and Allen (1983) have reported various "syndromes" of developmental language disorders associating each with a specific profile of speech-language abilities and relating these profiles to underlying deficits in various brain areas. If the various disorders of speech-language development, including motor speech disorders, result from underlying dysfunction in neurolinguistic subsystems within the left hemisphere, supporting evidence should be available. The next section reviews information that implicates potential left- (and sometimes right-) hemisphere deficits as a contributing factor in certain developmental speech-language and other learning disorders.

Deviations in Neurologic Development that Might Contribute to Motor Speech Disorders

The processes of proliferation, migration, and differentiation result in the formation of various neurologic functional subsystems. These processes may be disrupted by a variety of factors including genetic deviations, toxic agents, and/or disease (Risser & Edgell, 1988). The extent and timing of the disruption plays a significant role in determining functional consequences. It is possible that less pronounced disruptions occurring in the developing brain may result in more subtle neuroanatomic malformations such as abnormal dendritic growth, arrested myelination, or other cellular deformities. This possibility implicates a congenital, possibly genetic, neurologic etiology for developmental motor speech disorders. The historical review in Chapter 1 contains many implications for a congenital, genetic, neurologically based deficit: More males are involved; there is more left-handedness or mixed laterality; there have been documented family pedigrees; and there is a strong association with other developmental learning disabilities. If children demonstrate developmental motor speech disorders as a result of congenital (possibly genetic) disruptions in neurologic maturation, then why do we only infrequently find confirming signs of neurologic abnormality? The answer to this question may reflect the type of neurologic deviations contributing to speech-language as well as related learning disabilities. Neurologic differences need not produce "hard signs" of neurological damage. In short, different is not necessarily abnormal. Geschwind (1979) discussed the concept of "an alternative type of anatomical variation as a causal factor in defective acquisition of language skills" (p. 146). His proposals stem from a genetic disposition and assume that each individual demonstrates limitations in various skill areas. He suggested that limitations (and strengths) portray genetic variation among individuals and that behavioral deviations, such as speech-language deficits, may be direct reflections of neuroanatomical alterations. This position has received support from studies of brain-behavior relationships addressing the biological bases of various learning disabilities. At least two related bodies of information merit consideration: imaging studies and anatomical studies.

Imaging Studies: Windows to the Brain

Hier, Lemay, Rosenberger, and Perlo (1978) analyzed computerized brain tomograms (CT scans) of 24 individuals with developmental dyslexia for evidence of cerebral asymmetry. The usual pattern of asymmetry (in right-handed people) is for the left-hemisphere language areas, such as the temporal planum and perisylvian cortex (Galaburda, LeMay, Kemper, & Geschwind, 1978) and frontal operculum (Wada, Clarke, & Hamm, 1975), to be visibly larger than corresponding areas in the right hemisphere. In the Hier et al. study, 10 subjects presented a reversal of this pattern in the parietooccipital region (R > L). These 10 individuals had a lower mean verbal IQ than the remaining 14 patients, and 4 of the 10 presented a history of delayed speech-language development (defined as the onset of phrases after 3 years). Only 1 of the other 14 cases displayed a history of delayed speech-language development. The authors interpreted this rather high percentage of reversed asymmetry among dyslexic brains as suggesting "that a variant pattern of cerebral asymmetry may be a factor contributing to the reading disability of certain individuals" (p. 90). The 40% (4 of 10) rate of delayed speech-language development in the brains with reversed asymmetry might suggest that patterns of hemispheric asymmetry may be related to variations of verbal language development as well as written language development. This apparent association should not surprise many researchers or clinicians.

A later study by Haslam, Dalby, Johns, and Rademaker (1981) challenged some of the findings reported by Hier and colleagues. These investigators did not find a high proportion of reversed asymmetry among dyslexic specimens; however, they did find a high proportion of hemisphere symmetry (L = R). Six of their subjects presented a history of speech-language delay (here defined as the failure to use two-word utterances by 2 years or simple sentences by 3 years). Of these six, one had reversed asymmetry, one was symmetrical, and four presented the expected asymmetry pattern.

The discrepancies between the results of the Hier and Haslam studies may relate to the type of subjects studied by each group of investigators. The subjects studied by Hier et al. were considerably older than those studied by Haslam's group and 25% were left-handed compared to 100% right-handed in the Haslam study. Age alone should not contribute to the observed differences in hemispheric asymmetry (the proportion of hemispheric asymmetries is similar in children and adults according to Wada, Clarke, & Hamm, 1975), but handedness may have been a contributing factor (LeMay, 1977). Results from a study by Parkins, Roberts, Reinarz, and Varney (1987), suggested that asymmetry among right-handed dyslexics was similar to controls, whereas left-handed dyslexics demonstrated significant variations from the expected pattern of L > R.

Although these studies differed with respect to their specific observations, they were in agreement that "abnormal" patterns of hemispheric asymmetry (reversed or symmetrical) may be associated with developmental dyslexia. This pattern seems most pronounced among left-handed individuals and among dyslexics with a history of speech-language deficits. Given that these studies did not identify any significant evidence of brain damage, their findings implicate substantial variation among gross neuroanatomy (specifically hemispheric size relations) in brains of individuals demonstrating written and/or spoken language deficits.

More recently, Plante, Swisher, Vance, and Rapcsak (1991) investigated variations in hemispheric morphology in children with specific language impairment. Similar to the findings in dyslexic brains (especially those with a history of speech-language deficits), magnetic resonance imaging (MRI) scans in boys with specific language impairment revealed atypical perisylvian asymmetries. This observation led the authors to suggest that "a prenatal alteration of brain development underlies specific language impairment" (p. 52). Although no mention was made of these boys' reading abilities, it is interesting to note that three of the eight boys had reported family histories of dyslexia.

In a companion study, Plante (1991) reported that parents and siblings of boys with specific language impairment, especially those in families with a history of speech-language deficits, demonstrated atypical perisylvian asymmetries. This observation was inferred to indicate a "transmittable, biological factor that places some families at risk for language impairment" (p. 67).

Written and spoken language impairments share many common features. Atypical organization of the cerebral hemispheres may be such a feature, especially when a family history of difficulty with these abilities is present. More often that not in these cases, observed asymmetries are believed to reflect some type of "underdevelopment" of the left hemisphere.

Anatomical Studies: Microscopic Deviations

The presence of frequent deviations in hemispheric size relations in the absence of evidence for gross neuroanatomic damage suggests anatomic deviations at a more microscopic level. It has long been known that deviations in brain morphology are prominent in retarded individuals (Crome, 1960); however, it was not until a case report by Drake (1968) that less obvious anatomic deviations were associated with various learning disabilities. In postmortem examination of a brain obtained from a dyslexic individual, Drake observed abnormal parietal gyri bilaterally along with irregularities in the corpus callosum and subcortical white matter. These patterns of anatomic deviations were not attributed to brain damage. Rather, they were believed to reflect disrupted cellular migration during fetal development. Despite historical significance and importance in understanding brain-behavior relationships underlying language deficits, Drake's findings were not duplicated until 11 years later. Galaburda and his colleagues (Galaburda & Eidelberg, 1982; Galaburda & Kemper, 1979) reported gross anatomical and cytoarchitectonic abnormalities in the brain of a 19-year-old male who had been diagnosed as dyslexic at the age of 5. Extensive clinical history was available for their subject making this case particularly important in studying brain-language relationships.

Galaburda's Case

Description. The subject was born at term with no prenatal or perinatal complications. He was the youngest of four siblings. Early development was judged normal except he was noted to be clumsier than his siblings. Speech was delayed in that sentences did not emerge until after 3 years. No further speech-language details were reported. Reading and spelling difficulties were noted in elementary school. The first grade was repeated, and at that time, a diagnosis of developmental dyslexia was made. Routine neurological exam revealed no abnormalities, and his IQ (Stanford-Binet) was in the normal range. This pattern persisted into high school where, in addition to reading and spelling problems, difficulties were identified in arithmetic skills, right-left orientation, and finger localization. Dichotic listening tests revealed marked right-ear superiority (left hemisphere control of auditory language). Nocturnal seizures developed at age 16, but were controlled with medication. At this time neurological exam, EEG, and isotope scan were considered normal. The patient was left-handed and his father and both brothers were slow readers, but not his mother or sister.

Anatomical Deviations.   On visual inspection the brain presented neither gross abnormalities nor signs of trauma. The hemispheres were asymmetrical (L > R), and no irregularities were observed in the subcortical white matter, basal ganglia, brainstem, cerebellum, or corpus callosum. The temporal planum was not asymmetrical, but rather described as "approximately equal" in both hemispheres. Under microscopic inspection, multiple abnormalities were observed in the left hemisphere. The most pronounced deviation was an area of micropolygyria (many small gyri) confined to the posterior portion of Heschl's gyrus and the temporal plane. In addition, mild areas of focal dysplasia (abnormal tissue) were noted throughout the left hemisphere—primarily in the parietal, occipital, and temporal lobes with a large collection of these deviations in the inferior parietal lobule (usually defined as the supramarginal and angular gyri). By far, the greatest amount of cellular deviation was noted in the language areas within the left hemisphere.

Implications for Speech-Language Disorders.   Two of the findings from Galaburda's case have important implications for studying neurologic form in reference to speech-language abilities. The area of the temporal plane was bilaterally symmetrical, a pattern not seen in other hemisphere areas from this brain. This observation might be taken as "a sign of congenital deviation in cerebral organization that favors the occurrences of delayed speech" (Geschwind, 1979, p. 151). Also, morphological deviance at the cellular level may relate to speech-language and reading difficulties. Kemper (1982) presented a second case in which less extensive anatomical deviations were noted—along with a less severe form of dyslexia. Galaburda, Sherman, Rosen, Aboitz, and Geschwind (1985) reported cortical abnormalities in four consecutive cases (including the one described above), all of which demonstrated left-hemisphere irregularities in areas felt to subserve language functions.

The relationship between these anatomical findings and speech-language development deviations is speculative at best. The studies include only a few subjects and were designed to study potential neurologic bases of dyslexia.

They provided very limited details of speech-language performance. However, the findings of these investigations do implicate structural abnormalities in the left-hemisphere language areas in brains of individuals with developmental speech-language deficits as well as dyslexia. These findings occur in the absence of overt signs of neurologic deficit.

Collectively, imaging and anatomic studies implicate a difference in the development of the left hemisphere among individuals with speech-language and reading difficulties. Until recently, these studies have under-emphasized the role of spoken language; however, the frequent relationship between written and spoken language deficits forces similar neurologic considerations on the search for explanation of a biologic cause of severe speech-language disorders in children. An hypothesis might be formulated to state that children with speech-language disorders demonstrate differences in left-hemisphere development, specifically within areas felt to subserve speech-language functions. Because we envision the left hemisphere to function in "subsystems" in performing various speech-language tasks, we might hypothesize further that anatomic deviations in different areas within the left hemisphere would contribute to different patterns of speech-language deficit.

Following a subsystems' approach, it would be logical that certain behaviors using the same subsystem would be "related" and that by virtue of their relationship might show clinical commonalities. Among children with developmental motor speech disorders there seems to be a special relationship among motor, speech-language, and reading abilities. This clinical observation would suggest that these functions use, at least to some degree, the same neurologic subsystems. From a developmental perspective, it is obvious that many children "outgrow" overt speech problems and that many of them seem to develop new problems—dyslexia being prominent among these. These clinical observations give rise to basic questions that bear on our neurolinguistic subsystems concept: (1) Why do some children outgrow developmental motor speech deficits and why do others persist? and (2) Why do other, presumably related, problems, emerge?

The Illusion of the Vanishing Disorder

It is obvious that every child with speech production deficits does not retain those deficits into adulthood. It would be wonderful to attribute such progress to the benefits of education or speech-language therapy, but this position cannot explain all of the children who persist with disorders despite intensive, appropriate treatment. Furthermore, if deficient neurologic subsystems are responsible for certain developmental motor speech disorders, one must consider that other subsystems are utilized to develop more "normal" speech abilities. These positions lead to some interesting questions regarding developing neurologic systems and the acquisition of skills in the presence of neurologic dysfunction. Earlier in this chapter the question was raised: "Is there more than one way to learn how to speak?" From a subsystems perspective the answer is "yes"—but that "other way of speaking" should have some predictable differences (McCarthy & Warrington, 1984). In this regard, children with developmental motor speech disorders (as well as other speech-language deficits) would be expected to have the capacity to change over time to "hide" their limitations, possibly by way of compensatory, alternate speech-language or other strategies.

Chameleons and Compensations

Speech is a social behavior. Not only do children use speech to communicate with their environment, the environment also influences the characteristics of speech used by the child. Peters (1977) has asserted that different language processing strategies can be identified in children learning to communicate verbally. Furthermore, she contended that children with speech-language difficulties may differ from children with normal speech-language abilities in the repertoire of strategies available to them. Weeks (1974) described a child who had limited strategies for learning language, but who was adept at using other learning strategies in compensation of language limitations. Most clinicians have observed change in communicative (including speech) behavior that is not treatment related. For example, children who enter kindergarten with a fluent, unintelligible style of speech and leave with a nonfluent, more intelligible, but still defective style of speech. The observations of change over time and the influence of the child's environment raise interesting questions regarding interactions between neurologic maturation/function and environmental influences.

Earlier in this chapter possible roles of the right hemisphere in speech-language functioning were discussed. It is not inconceivable that the right hemisphere retains certain speech-language functions in instances in which the left hemisphere is maturationally and/or structurally unprepared to perform them. The most dramatic example of this potential situation is the case of left hemisphere removal early in childhood. However, clinicians reading the depiction of right-hemisphere language functions reviewed earlier in this chapter would certainly recognize many children who have displayed developmental speech-language deficits, including some with developmental motor speech disorders.

Another possible, not necessarily discrepant position, is that deviations in left-hemisphere development facilitate the development of alternative left-hemisphere subsystems to perform speech-language activities. At least two possibilities may be considered. In individuals with anomalous cortical growth (e.g., that reported in Galaburda's series of brains of dyslexic individuals), the deviant cortex may establish connections with other, appropriate cortical systems to form a functional, albeit impaired, speech-language system (see Chapter

8 in Finger & Stein, 1982 for relevant discussion). It is also possible that cortical areas adjacent to deviant cortex may subsume some of the functions mediated by the impaired areas (Chapters 8 and 15 in Finger & Stein, 1982).

Each of these possibilities relates to Luria's (1980) reorganization model. Luria felt that any functional act was an element of a larger behavioral system. If part of that system was impaired (e.g., damaged or underdeveloped), the system would reorganize in an attempt to perform the functional act, perhaps in a different way. This position is not inconsistent with the neurolinguistic subsystems concept. The problem, at this time, is defining the nature of various subsystems. For now, models like those presented by Kent and McNeil (1987) and McCarthy and Warrington (1984) are valuable as conceptualizations of various clinical deficits and may be useful to explain changes in speech-language performance over time.

Why Do Some Problems Persist?

Most clinicians implicate severity as a factor in persistent problems. This is reflected in the descriptive writings of Worster-Drought and Morley (see Chapter 1) relevant to children with developmental motor speech disorders. The real question is "What determines severity?" From a neurobiological perspective one might assume that more severe speech-language problems result from larger "lesions." This certainly seems to apply when considering the extensive morphological deviations seen in retarded individuals (Crome, 1960) and in certain individuals with severe language deficits (Landau, Goldstein, & Kleffner, 1960). However, such reports also imply that larger "lesions" impair more than just speech-language functions. Thus, there are two possibilities to consider: (1) more disruption within speech-language functions, and (2) disruption to other "cognitive" functions that might impede development of speech-language systems.

Greater Impairment Within Speech-Language Functions

Bishop and Edmundson (1987) reported that prognosis in language impairment might be related to the pattern of language performance. Persisting deficits may be related directly to the range of language functions that are impaired. In studying correlates of severe and persistent speech-language disorders in children, Robinson (1991) reported that "these children rarely have a pure disorder affecting only one part of speech or language function" (p. 946).

Reports such as these suggest that children with more severe and/or diffuse speech-language deficits have a poorer prognosis for improvement. Although it would be difficult to argue with this position, it may be advisable to expand its perspective somewhat. Specifically, children with more severe speech-language deficits *may* have generally poor information processing skills and/or other, related impairments that (a) contribute to the impression of a more severe speech-language deficit and/or (b) function to impede further development (and/or compensation) of the speech-language system.

Impeding Processes

The cognitive demands associated with a speech-language task may influence the performance of the task. McNeil, Odell, and Tseng (1991) discussed an alternative conceptualization of acquired aphasia in adults focusing on allocation of cognitive resources. These authors consider aphasia in the framework of attentional mechanisms. They contend that each individual has a limited but flexible supply of attention. The individual may direct this attention proportionally to any task—including various aspects of speech-language processing. If one aspect of information processing requires an inordinately large amount of attention and/or the individual has difficulty allocating this cognitive resource, then other aspects of performance will be impaired. This occurs not because of a direct deficit in a specific task component, but because insufficient attention is available to provide proper cognitive support for that component. Given the same task in another cognitive environment, the individual may perform flawlessly or, at least, superiorly. This conceptual position does have support from studies of both adults and children with speech-language deficits. Tompkins and Flowers (1985) demonstrated that increasing cognitive demands on a task of perception of emotional intonation interfered with some adult subjects' ability to perform the task. Specifically, patients with left-hemisphere damage performed similarly to normal controls at simple task levels. However, their performance deteriorated dramatically when cognitive demands for the perception task were increased. LaPointe and Erickson (1991) reported a similar pattern in a study of auditory processing abilities in adults with aphasia. They studied the effects of divided attention on auditory vigilance (simply stated, listening for a specific auditory target) and reported that, when adults with aphasia were required to perform dual tasks simultaneously, their ability to correctly identify auditory targets was significantly reduced.

Campbell and McNeil (1985) demonstrated that manipulating cognitive demands influenced task performance in children. These investigators demonstrated that altering attention requirements had a beneficial effect on auditory comprehension tasks performed by children with language impairments. Following Kahneman's (1973) information processing model Campbell and McNeil suggested that these children, who had suffered brain damage related to convulsive disorder, had limited but not fixed attentional capacity. They felt that the task demands would determine how the children would allocate this resource. By lowering attentional demands on an initial comprehension task, Campbell and McNeil were able to facilitate improved comprehension on a subsequent task.

Reports such as these suggest that cognitive demands of a task may en-hance or impair performance of that task. This might imply the presence of a limited set of available resources. If a child is allocating substantial resources to one function (e.g., speech production), other functions may be performed more poorly. Likewise, it is possible that if a child is "focusing" on a specific component of a complex task (e.g., motor aspect of speech production), then other aspects might be performed at an inferior level. In instances where tasks demands are less, the overall performance would be expected to improve. Children with more severe speech-language deficits may have to allocate cog-nitive resources more widely to be able to perform communicative tasks. It is conceivable that this situation might lead to slower acquisition of new skills related to speech-language function.

Relevant to children with motor speech disorders, the child must contend with a limited motor system in addition to speech-language limitations. In se-vere cases both of these deficits may be persistent. Robinson (1991) report-ed that 90% of his sample of children with severe, persistent speech-language disorders had significant motor impairments (in this case meaning "clumsi-ness" in the absence of hard neuromotor deficits). Although nothing is proved via anecdotal correlations, the possibility should be considered that the dis-persion of deficits in these children may have required a substantial amount of other cognitive resources just to perform speech-language tasks at an im-paired level.

Why Do Other Problems Emerge?

Speaking and Reading

A striking clinical relationship exists between speech-language disorders and dyslexia. This is evident from the historical review presented in Chapter 1 and from the information in this chapter. Catts (1989) has pointed out that language disorders underlie most cases of developmental dyslexia. He postu-lated that phonological processing deficits may underlie many of the prob-lems seen in dyslexia. Furthermore, he suggested (Catts, 1986) that the phon-ological processing deficits seen in dyslexics also may contribute to speech production errors in these children. Specifically, he suggested that difficulty in the "planning" stage of speech production might account for some of the speech production deficits observed in dyslexic children. Catts (1989) noted that some aspects of speech production in dyslexics (i.e., slow rate) might re-flect limitations in motor processes, although the majority of speech errors were attributed to deficits in phonological planning rather than motor execution.

The observations of Catts and many clinicians and researchers before him are not surprising. A neurological and a linguistic relationship appears to exist between spoken and written language. Models of reading functions often include parallels to speaking functions (Margolin, 1984). Error patterns in various types of dyslexia (Marshall & Newcombe, 1973; Shallice & Warrington, 1975) have been explained in similar fashion to different types of speech deficits (McCarthy & Warrington, 1984). In this respect, it is not surprising that many children demonstrating severe speech-language problems, especially those with deficient phonologic development, demonstrate difficulties with written language later on. Because children with developmental motor speech disorders demonstrate some form of phonological deficit, they would be expected to be at significant risk for subsequent identification of dyslexia. Given some of Catts' (1986, 1989) observations, it would not be unexpected to learn that the patterns of reading and speaking deficits had some degree of similarity.

Phoneme-Grapheme Conversion: Spelling Problems

Snowling and Stackhouse (1983) studied spelling and reading performance in four children considered to demonstrate developmental apraxia of speech. Performances of the children with apraxia of speech were compared to a group of children with normal speech abilities matched for reading level. The children with apraxia of speech were inferior to the normal-speaking group on spelling and reading tasks. The authors interpreted their results to indicate that the children with apraxia of speech had more difficulty with phonetic spelling strategies and were less adept at phoneme-grapheme conversions. They suggested that their spelling difficulties were not the result of poor articulation nor poor knowledge of letter forms. Rather, they posited that the children with apraxia of speech had difficulty with speech-sound analysis at a level prior to phoneme-grapheme conversion. This position sounds remarkably similar to Catts' (1989) suggestion of a deficit in phonological planning for speech in certain dyslexic children. Snowling and Stackhouse (1983) suggested that this type of reading deficit would create a reliance on "sight vocabulary" in reading tasks. This type of reading deficit (deep dyslexia) implies direct access from visual input into a semantic analyzer (Colheart, 1980). As such, Snowling and Stackhouse (1983) are implying that children with developmental apraxia of speech may demonstrate impaired phonologic processing with preserved semantic analysis. This reflects one of the "routes" of speech production described by McCarthy and Warrington (1984). Based on this comparison, it is conceivable that phonological aspects of reading and speaking in children with developmental apraxia of speech might be improved by enhancing the semantic components of the respective tasks. Although this provides for interesting speculation, the study by Snowling and Stackhouse (1983) does not directly address the issue of apraxia as a motor speech disorder, other than to consider apraxic speakers as a subgroup of children with severe phonological disorders.

Motor Dysfunctions and Dyslexia

Studies by Wolff, Michel, and Ovrut (1990) and Byring and Pulliainen (1984) speak more directly to the relatedness of motor dysfunctions and dyslexia. Wolff et al. (1990) found that dyslexic adolescents and adults were slower on tasks of nonsense syllable repetition than normal readers and learning disabled adolescents without dyslexia. In dyslexic adolescents, motor speech deficits (slow rate and sequencing errors) correlated moderately, but significantly with performance on standardized tests of reading ability. Byring and Pulliainen (1984) compared 34 adults with poor spelling ability and 34 controls on an extensive neuropsychological battery including reading, writing, language, and motor tasks. Results revealed a pattern of deficient left-hemisphere information processing. The poor spelling group was inferior to the control subjects on a variety of fine motor tasks, phoneme manipulation tasks (location of a target phoneme in a word, phonemic synthesis), and nonverbal auditory tasks (perception of rhythmic sequences). Byring and Pulliainen (1984) concluded that the pattern of deficiencies noted in the poor spelling subjects "may be due to incomplete development of the analytic-sequential skills generally attributed to the left hemisphere" (p. 771).

Findings from various studies implicate a defective phonologic processor as a variable in certain types of dyslexia. Children with developmental motor speech disorders demonstrate deficient phonologic processing. Dyslexic children and adults demonstrate subtle motor deficits. These observations do not implicate motor or motor speech dysfunction as the direct cause of phonologically based dyslexias. Rather, they suggest that children with developmental motor speech disorders may later demonstrate dyslexia, presumably secondary to a persistent phonological disorder. From this perspective it would be interesting to observe whether different types of motor deficits would predict different types of phonologic impairments leading to different types of dyslexic deficits. Such a study has not been completed.

Implications and Considerations

The neurolinguistic perspective offered in this chapter is incomplete. No doubt more pieces will be added to the puzzle by further research and case study. The facts are that some children with speech-language impairments and/or dyslexia demonstrate non-brain-damage variations on anatomical and/or imaging (CT, MRI) indices of hemisphere anatomy. Although these findings along with clinical observations of relationships among motor speech, language, and reading performances tempt readers to subscribe to the left-hemisphere deficit hypothesis, this is not a proven phenomenon. It would be erroneous to assume that all children with these clinical disorders had anatomical deviations within the left hemisphere. Nonetheless, there are striking clinical similarities among motor, speech-language, and reading performances in *some* children. A common link seems to be the developing phonological system. In the next chapter, a "motolinguistic" model will be presented that attempts to organize a perspective on potential relationships between motor and speech-language functions with consideration for deviant phonological performance.

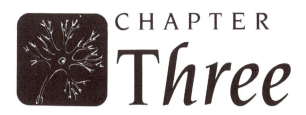

CHAPTER

Three

A Motolinguistic Perspective

Meaningful speech is a motor phenomenon that is dependent on linguistic input. In some instances both motor and linguistic processes are disrupted in the same individual. This scenario raises important questions for the study of developmental motor speech disorders. At least two questions must be addressed to better understand the potential for a motolinguistic basis for developmental motor speech disorders: (1) What is the relationship between nonspeech motor ability and speech ability relating to left-hemisphere control, and (2) Is there evidence of motor "subsystems" that parallel speech-language subsystems within the left hemisphere?

Motor and Speech Relations Controlled by the Left Hemisphere

Historically, relations between nonspeech oral motor performance and speech ability have been related to findings in adults who have suffered left-hemisphere damage. Poor performance in voluntary nonspeech oral motor tasks such as sticking out the tongue or puffing the cheeks following left-hemisphere damage has been described since Jackson (1878/1932) and is typically attributed to some form of apraxia (De Renzi, Pieczuro, & Vignolo, 1966; Nathan, 1947). In certain aphasic individuals these nonspeech motor deficits coexist with speech production deficits, thus providing an observable, clinical relationship between the two functions.

One Master Control or Many Related Subsystems?

Kimura (1976) felt that these functions were related to each other and to control of voluntary hand movement (i.e., gestures) to such a degree that she hypothesized a common neural system (or systems) within the dominant hemisphere responsible for coordination of finely controlled movements. Studies of adults with left-hemisphere lesions by Kimura (1978), Mateer and Kimura (1977), and Kimura and Watson (1989) have implicated a common or related system underlying speech and nonspeech facial movements. Patients with right-hemisphere lesions did not demonstrate these observed relationships (Mateer, 1978). Mateer and Dodrill (unpublished, cited in Mateer, 1983) used the WADA test (anesthetization of a cerebral hemisphere via intracarotid injection of sodium amytal) to evaluate relations between speech articulation and nonspeech facial movement in the right and left hemispheres of right-handed adults. They observed simultaneous disruption of both functions with left-hemisphere injection, but no disruption following right-hemisphere injection. Ojemann and Mateer (1979) used a cortical stimulation paradigm to study relations among nonspeech facial movement and various speech and language tasks. In this paradigm, areas of cortex are stimulated with electric current simultaneously with a request to perform a task (e.g., facial movement, speech, auditory perception). The electric current acts to impair the normal function of the area being stimulated. Thus, if an abnormal response is obtained with stimulation to a specific cortical area, it is assumed that the stimulated area has some role in the performance of the experimental task. Using this task, Ojemann and Mateer found such a high degree of overlap in left-hemisphere cortical areas related to nonspeech facial movement and speech articulation they hypothesized that the two functions were part of the same cortical system.

Evidence in Children

Demonstration of this relationship in children has been less pronounced. However, indications exist that speech/nonspeech motor functions may have a common control system within the left hemisphere. Recall Simonds and Schiebel's (1989) findings regarding neuromaturation of motor and speech areas. Development of primary motor control areas precedes development of motor speech areas, but with maturation, the motor speech areas dominate between 2 and 3 years of age. Thus, there seems to be a temporal link between nonspeech and speech neural systems from the beginning. A technique called "time-sharing" has been used to study left- versus right-hemisphere control of speech-language functions in both normal and speech-language impaired children. Basically, the theory behind this technique is that two functions that use the same neural systems will compete for use of that system when the functions are performed at the same time (review Chapter 2, resource allocation theory). If two functions sharing the same system are performed at the same time, one of the functions will show a deterioration in performance. This phenomenon has been demonstrated between speech and nonspeech motor functions both in normal-speaking children (Kinsbourne & McMurray, 1975; Piazza, 1977) and children with speech-language disorders (Hughes & Sussman, 1983).

In summary, a variety of investigational techniques in both adults and children have implicated a neurologic relationship between nonspeech oral movements and speech production. These functions seem to be controlled by a system or systems within the left hemisphere.

Evidence for Nonspeech and Speech Subsystems within the Left Hemisphere

Aphasia and Apraxia of Speech in Adults

In adults, following lesions to the left hemisphere, there is evidence for "selective" impairment to motor and motor speech systems. Most clinicians are familiar with the obvious motoric struggle in the speech of patients with Broca's aphasia. This pattern, referred to by some researchers as apraxia of speech, traditionally has been associated with anterior lesions within the left hemisphere. Conversely, individuals demonstrating aphasia-related speech deficits in the absence of obvious motoric struggle frequently demonstrate more posterior lesions within the left hemisphere. At a superficial level this apparent dichotomy makes sense. Anterior regions within the hemisphere, including frontal and anterior parietal, form the origin of the descending motor pathways. Damage to these areas would be expected to contribute to observable motor deficits. Yet, the observed motor and speech dysfunctions do not reflect paralysis or paresis caused by damage to direct motor systems. Rather, these motor/speech abnormalities often are observed situationally. That is, the same oral structures perform certain motor tasks without impairment while other motor functions are severely impaired. This pattern of motor behavior typically is referred to as apraxia. There is evidence from at least two sources suggesting that lesions in the anterior versus posterior aspects of the left hemisphere will produce different types of motor impairments or apraxias.

Differential Motor Impairment in Apraxia: Clinicoanatomical Evidence

Tognola and Vignolo (1980) compared lesion location (identified by CT scan) and oral apraxia in adults with left hemisphere lesions. Using single oral movements as their oral motor task, they reported that, within the left hemisphere, the inferior frontal cortex and juxtaposed areas of the superior temporal gyrus and insula were important in determining presence of oral apraxia. Mateer and Kimura (1977) reported that nonfluent aphasic subjects (anterior left-hemisphere lesions) demonstrated deficits in both single oral movements and sequences of oral movements, whereas subjects with fluent aphasia (posterior left-hemisphere lesions) demonstrated deficits primarily in the production of oral movement sequences. These observations suggest steps, levels, or subsystems in the performance of oral movements relative to left-hemisphere control. Posterior regions are inferred to govern the selection and ordering of movement sequences; anterior regions are inferred to be responsible for the execution of both single movements and movement sequences.

The same pattern of anterior-posterior control for oral movements was identified by Ojemann and Mateer (1979) using a cortical stimulation paradigm. These investigators reported that cortical disruption by electrical stimulation in the posterior inferior frontal lobe (just anterior to the face motor area on the primary motor strip) impaired production of single movements and movement sequences. Preservation of single movements with impaired movement sequences was observed following stimulation to some areas of inferior frontal cortex, but was much more prominent in superior temporal and parietal areas. These data, as well as those obtained from studies of adults with brain damage, suggest that posterior left-hemisphere subsystems within speech-language cortex govern the selection, ordering, and organization of oral movement sequences, whereas anterior subsystems govern the execution of both single and sequential movements. These implied patterns are depicted in Figure 3–1. These patterns of oral movement breakdown appear to parallel impairments in speech production seen in aphasic adults. In fact, Kimura and Watson (1989) reported striking similarities between speech and nonspeech oral movement performances in adults with left-anterior versus left-posterior lesions. They reported further that left-hemisphere damaged patients without speech-language impairment (nonaphasic) did not perform differently from right-hemisphere damaged patients. Neither group made substantial errors on the respective tasks. They concluded that oral movement control is closely tied to speech motor control.

Subsystems of Speech and Motor Control

Motor Control

The execution of any motor behavior may follow a similar path. Motor behavior starts with a goal or idea which is organized into a plan, coded into a specific motor program, and executed. Brooks (1986) described these activities in reference to potential systems of neural regulation. From an emotive base the limbic system demands movement. Activity in association cortex

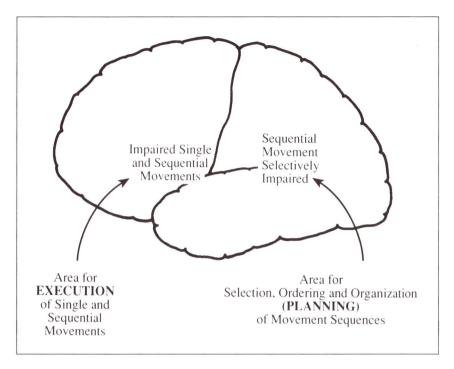

Figure 3–1. Left-hemisphere areas involved in the execution of single and sequential movements and the selection, ordering, and organization of movement sequences.

(e.g., prefrontal, parietal, and temporal) analyzes these demands and formulates a strategy or plan of action. This plan is forwarded to projection cortex, which in combination with various subcortical and brainstem structures formulates specific motor tactics or programs that are to be executed.

Motor Speech Control

In favorable circumstances, speech production begins with an idea. To communicate this idea, the speaker must organize it into a linguistic code that contains meaning (semantics) and form (syntax). The form of the message then must be shaped into units of speech production. These units must be organized according to their own rules of appropriate combination (phonology). Because speech is a "physical phenomenon," these organized speech units must be transformed or coded into a motor program. Subsequently, this motor program is used to execute movements of the vocal tract that result in production of the organized speech units. In this framework, depicted in Figure 3–2, speech begins as a mental concept that becomes linguistically organized, is transformed into motor behavior, and is executed as movement. Activity at any step along the process will influence the next step and possibly the preceding step.

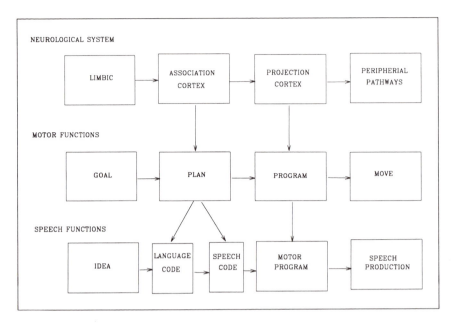

Figure 3-2. Parallel organization of motor and speech functions from concept to movement.

Admittedly, this is a simplified version of a complex process. The primary points to consider are: (1) There is evidence that speech-language and non-speech motor functions overlap within the left hemisphere, and (2) There seems to be a division of labor within the left hemisphere that pertains to both speech and nonspeech functions such that posterior areas are responsible for selection of movement targets and ordering of sequential targets, and anterior areas seem to govern formation of motor programs for all motor behaviors. As demonstrated in models such as that presented by Kent and McNeil (1987; see Chapter 2), there are many potential information processing steps applicable to speech production between the selection of targets and the execution of movement. From this perspective, we can hypothesize that there will be different types of speech/motor breakdowns depending on which component of the controlling system is impaired.

Differential Patterns of Motor/Speech Breakdown: The Apraxias

Historical Perspectives

It is important to ascertain at the outset of this discussion that the focus of motor disorders to be discussed does not include disorders that are the direct result of paresis or paralysis in the motor system. At issue is the differential pattern of motor and motor speech deficits associated with presumed cortical disruptions in the overlapping speech-language and motor systems within the left hemisphere. Variations among motor deficits of this nature have long been recognized as variants of apraxia. Geschwind (1975) in his classic paper on the "apraxias" emphasized that apraxia is not a unitary disorder—there are multiple variants. Preceding Geschwind, description of apraxia variants abounded in historical literature. The German neurologist Liepmann is generally credited with the initial delineation of the apraxias (Hecaen & Albert, 1978). Although the terms used to described these variants have changed with passing time, the differentiating characteristics have remained quite consistent. Ideational apraxia is regarded as an impairment or loss of the concept of a complex movement. Traditionally associated with posterior lesions (parieto-occipital), this variant is most often seen as an impairment in performance of a complex action requiring two or more objects. Ideomotor apraxia is envisioned as an impairment in the organization of a motor act. Associated with parietal areas (supramarginal, arcuate fasciculus, and posterior perisylvian), this subtype of apraxia was viewed as a dissociation between the idea of a movement and its motor execution. Melokinetic or limb-kinetic apraxia was associated with impairment in single movements. In this condition more complex movement sequences may not even get started. Associated with lesions in the precentral motor area, this type of apraxia was felt to be purely executive, resting somewhere between paresis and apraxia.

Roy's Refinement

Many anatomic and functional depictions of apraxic disorders have been offered over the years. A interesting summary and reanalysis of apraxic variants was presented by Roy (1978). Roy proposed a categorization of apraxias "according to the basic underlying element in the functional system of skilled motor activity thought to be involved" (p. 191). He proposed three main categories: planning, executive, and unit apraxia. These variants are anatomically depicted in Figure 3–3.

Planning apraxia has two variants. Primary planning apraxia is associated with frontal lobe dysfunction resulting in some form of cognitive deficit. This variant of apraxia reflects deficits in any planning activity. Secondary planning apraxia is associated with parietal-occipital dysfunction resulting in a more general disturbance in spatial orientation. There is no associated general cognitive planning deficit. Executive apraxia results from damage to the premotor area. Individuals with this type of problem are expected to be able to plan movements but not execute them appropriately. There are no associated deficits as with planning apraxias. Unit apraxia represents a disorder in the "execution of individual movements with a sequence" (p. 198). It is associated with precentral and/or postcentral sensorimotor involvement. Al-

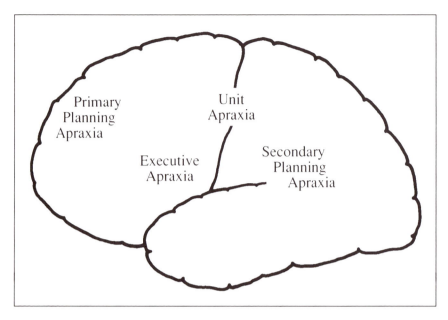

Figure 3–3. Neuroanatomic depiction of apraxia variants after Roy (1978).

though these descriptions are brief, they support the position that there are observable variants of motor deficits associated with dysfunction along an anterior-posterior dimension within the left-hemisphere system where motor and speech-language functions overlap.

From Hand to Mouth

The above descriptions of apraxic variants are related primarily to deficits in limb function, not to oral or speech movement deficits. However, there are precedents along these dimensions regarding speech and nonspeech oral motor deficits. Traditional views on speech fluency along an anterior-posterior dimension within the left hemisphere implicate different motor speech abilities associated with anterior versus posterior lesions. The parallels between oral motor performance and speech functions further implicate differential oral praxis and motor speech impairments along this left-hemisphere anterior-posterior dimension. Unfortunately, there has been little recognition of these experimental and/or clinical variants as they may pertain to oral and/or speech functions. For example, the term "apraxia of speech" that has become so frequently used implies a single variant as do the terms oral apraxia, buccofacial apraxia, and nonverbal facial apraxia. Within these "anatomic variants" of apraxia there is little recognition of "functional variation." In the final section of this chapter, a simplified model is offered that attempts to consider overlap between oral motor and speech functions and the operation of functional subsystems pertaining to both oral motor and speech functions within the left hemisphere.

A Proposed "Motolinguistic" Model of Cortical Motor Speech Disorders

The following model (Figure 3–4) represents an attempt to accommodate relationships between oral motor and motor speech deficits and clinical variants within each function. With specific reference to developmental motor speech disorders, there are at least two simple "position statements" that the model attempts to accommodate:

Position Statement 1

Overlapping motor and speech-language functions exist within the left-hemisphere "language areas."

Implication. Although motor and speech dysfunctions may occur independently, there are cases in which dysfunctions in both may occur.

Figure 3–4. A proposed motolinguistic model for developmental motor speech disorders.

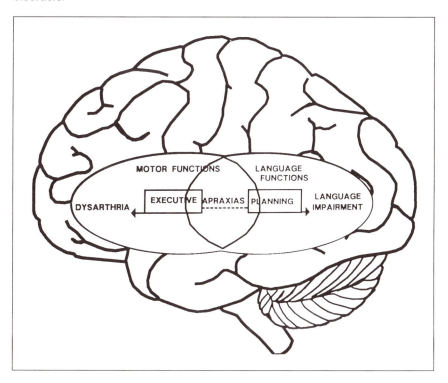

In these cases, the simultaneous dysfunctions are felt to be interrelated, not simply coexisting.

Position Statement 2

Along an anterior-posterior dimension within the left hemisphere there are various steps or levels in information processing that pertain both to motor and speech-language functions.

Implication. When simultaneous motor and speech deficits occur, the pattern of dysfunction in both will be similar.

A Continuum of Motor and Language Functions

Motolinguistic functions are envisioned along the anterior-posterior dimension as a continuum from executive functions to planning functions. There is no attempt to identify functions with specific neuroanatomical structures. Rather, the model reflects the perspective that frontal areas are important for the more motoric/executive aspects of speech and/or oral movement while the posterior (temporal-parietal) areas are important for the more linguistic and/or "planning" aspects. For example, the inferior frontal lobe areas and the motor projection areas for the face are the final common path for the development and implementation of motor programs relative to both speech and nonspeech oral motor activity. This general area is felt to be responsible for the execution of movements. Deficits relating to dysfunction in this area would be considered executive deficits. The "purest" executive deficit would be dysarthria secondary to abnormal function within the primary motor system. This corresponds clinically with congenital suprabulbar paresis. This speech deficit is felt to be at the extreme motor execution end of the continuum. Conversely, posterior temporal and parietal regions are felt to be important for linguistic formulation in speech and for selection and ordering of complex serial movements in nonspeech oral movements. Deficits at the far posterior end of the continuum would not be expected to demonstrate significant motor speech impairments. Sequencing deficits might be seen on various motor/language tasks related to deficits in selection and serial ordering. Such communicative impairments might be classified as specific language impairment. Moving forward on the continuum would enter those areas where nondysarthric motor speech disorders, specifically apraxias of speech, might be expected. These disorders are depicted as occurring when motor and speech-language dysfunctions overlap. Motor speech disorders at the posterior end of the apraxia continuum would be expected to reflect impaired planning in both motor and speech-language functions. Planning, as used in this context, would reflect difficulty with longer, more complex sequences of speech and oral motor behavior. At the extreme end of the planning continuum, one might expect difficulty with selection and ordering of targets within a sequence. More anteriorly, but still within the planning domain, one might expect correct sequential ordering but impaired ability to perform sequences. This type of impairment might be differentiated from an executive impairment by evaluating ability to perform single movements because the model would predict that cases with executive dysfunction would have difficulty even with single movements.

Supporting Evidence from Studies of Children

Evidence in support of the concepts inherent in the motolinguistic model have been offered for adults, but there is limited direct evidence in support of this model as it pertains to developmental motor speech disorders. Perhaps some support may be found in a study by Frisch and Handler (1974). These investigators compared performances on the Reitan-Indiana Neuropsychological Test Battery for Children among normal speaking children, children with articulation problems dominated by substitution errors, and children with articulation problems dominated by omission errors. The omission group yielded profiles similar to adults with left cerebral dysfunction. More specifically, the authors suggested that the pattern of errors presented by the omission group resembled what Luria (1980) referred to as "kinesthetic motor aphasia." This would implicate an area of involvement in the inferior postrolandic area of the left hemisphere that Whitaker (1971) hypothesized was involved in the phonological component of spoken language (temporal-parietal perisylvian region). These children had apparent concomitant motor deficits. Frisch and Handler (1974) concluded that "none of the subjects had any gross difficulties in performing motor acts, but many of those classified as having omission disorders seemed to have difficulties in patterning their motor actions, and, therefore performed motor tasks at a lower level" (p. 461). This observation implies a relationship between motor deficits and a specific pattern of speech deficits, possibly linked by a dysfunction toward the planning end of the proposed model.

Another source of evidence might be clinical studies of subtypes of speech-language impairment. One such study fits nicely as it interprets clinical symptoms in reference to inferred underlying neurologic subsystems. Rapin and Allen (1983) divided children with communicative disorders into seven groups on the basis of clinical observation, longitudinal results of observation, and clinical testing. Two of the resultant groups relate to the proposed model because they imply deficit left-hemisphere speech-language processes and present concomitant oral motor impairment. Children classified by Rapin and Allen as "severe expressive syndrome with good comprehension" were depicted as mute or unintelligible but with good comprehension of spoken language. Children classified as "phonologic-syntactic syndrome" were depicted as more verbal than the other group but demonstrated severe phonologic disorder with syntactic limitations that were not considered to be simple developmental delays. The authors implicated frontal and/or temporal-parietal dysfunction in these two groups. This suggestion would be consistent with the proposed model. Children with severely limited speech output and spared language comprehension would be portrayed at the extreme executive end of the continuum. Children with more verbal output and expressive language deficits would be portrayed more toward the planning end. Using this classification scheme, Lou, Henriksen, and Bruhn (1984) completed regional cerebral blood flow (rCBF) studies on 14 children. rCBF is a technique which allows investigators to infer metabolic activity and hence deviations in function in cerebral areas. Children with severe expressive syndrome (described as verbal apraxia by Lou et al.) demonstrated abnormalities primarily in frontal lobe areas. Children with phonologic-syntactic syndrome demonstrated more diffuse abnormalities along an extended anterior-posterior dimension of perisylvian cortex.

An additional study of relevance, presented by Dewey and Kaplan (1992), investigated subtypes of developmental motor deficits in reference to academic and language abilities. Four subtypes were identified from a group of 51 children. Of these, two subgroups had difficulty with praxis (voluntary movement) and sequencing tasks. These two subgroups demonstrated the most impairment on tests of receptive language, reading, and spelling. Dewey and Kaplan interpreted their findings to suggest a close relationship between sequencing ability, certain praxis deficits, and language-based skills. In the present motolinguistic model, children with sequencing deficits in combination with language comprehension impairment would be placed toward the extreme posterior end of the continuum.

Despite limitations in the nature and interpretation of each of the studies mentioned, they do provide initial evidence that this simple motolinguistic model may have a certain utility in helping clinicians to better understand children with developmental motor speech disorders. Available literature pertaining to dysarthria and apraxia of speech in children makes no effort to characterize motor and speech deficits into a functional model.

Clinical Predictions of Speech and Motor Performance

The motolinguistic model described in this chapter offers a framework for evaluating concurrent motor/speech limitations. Given this framework, certain predictions regarding motor/speech performance may be made. An abbreviated list of clinical predictions is offered in Table 3–1 for the hypothetical child demonstrating executive versus planning dysfunctions.

Table 3–1. Summary of clinical predictions of "pure" types from the motolinguistic model.

	Dysarthria	Executive Apraxia	Planning Apraxia	Language Deficit
Oral Motor:				
Motor weakness	yes	no	no	no
Abnormal reflexes	yes	no	no	no
Vegetative deficits	yes	occasionally	no	no
Single movements	related to patterns of weakness	poor	intact	intact
Movement sequence	related to patterns of weakness	poorer than single movements	poor	poor sequencing
Speech Production				
Motoric effort	yes	yes	no	no
Diadochokinesis	slow	slow	AMR > SMR	sequencing deficits possible
Sound repertoire	errors related to patterns of weakness	limited	>Executive	extensive
Language Expression	variable	limited	>Executive: grammatical errors	deficient
Language Comprehension	no predicted deficit	no predicted deficit	variable with some degree of deficit	deficient

Executive Apraxias: The Anterior End of the Continuum

On tasks of oral motor performance, the "executive child" would be expected to have difficulty with certain single movements. This does not mean poor execution of all oral movements as performance of many simple single movements may be preserved. It is important to note that any observed movement breakdowns should be differentiated from those seen as the result of paresis/paralysis as in the dysarthric child. Sequential oral movements will be especially troublesome for the child with executive dysfunction.

Because the model predicts that speech/motor functions will demonstrate parallel (overlapping) impairments, various speech abilities would be expected to show limitations similar to the nonspeech deficits. Performance of speech diadochokinesis tasks by the executive child would show a global deficit. Alternate motion tasks (repetition of the same syllable) may be accomplished but would be expected to be performed slowly. Sequential motion tasks (repetition of different syllables) would be extremely difficult or impossible for these children. The observed repertoire of speech sounds produced by executive children would be expected to be significantly reduced, and speech would be expected to show obvious motoric struggle. The limitation in speech output may range from mute (with preserved ability to vocalize) to the ability to produce a restricted number of speech sounds correctly or incorrectly.

The severe limitation of speech production abilities would have an obvious negative influence on expressive language performance. However, unless limb motor functions are impaired, these children may reveal an extensive expressive language ability via gestures. Although the motolinguistic model does not directly address language comprehension abilities, indirect predictions are possible. If the posterior aspects of the speech-language system are responsible for understanding spoken language, the child with a "pure" executive dysfunction (anterior portion of the system) would not be expected to demonstrate significant language comprehension deficits. In the hypothetical case, language comprehension would be "normal" or certainly superior to language expression.

At the anterior end of the continuum, the executive child may be differentiated from the dysarthric child on several criteria. Children demonstrating dysarthria will demonstrate paresis or other signs of direct motor deficit in the oral mechanism. Typically, these children will have deficits in nonspeech oral functions such as eating and control of saliva. Abnormal reflexes may be observed. Speech would be expected to be slow and reveal persistent motor effort. These children would be expected to have a larger speech sound repertoire than executive children, and many of their speech errors may be related to specific patterns of oral weakness (i.e., lips, tongue, velum, etc.). Because the speech deficits are the direct result of motor weakness, language deficits would not be considered central to the motor speech disorder. However, it would not be unexpected to observe concomitant language deficits, especially in expression.

Planning Apraxias: The Posterior End of the Continuum

Apraxia of speech often is described by the words "motor planning deficit" without any clarification of what this label indicates. In the motolinguistic model, planning apraxias are characterized by a common profile of speech-language and motor abilities. The child with planning dysfunction would be expected to reveal a different clinical picture from children with disorders at the anterior end of the motolinguistic continuum. The "planning child" would have little difficulty with single oral movements, but would demonstrate decreased performance as the sequential complexity of any attempted oral movement increased. A similar performance would be seen on tasks of speech diadochokinesis. Alternate motion rates would be superior to sequential motion rates and may be within normal limits. As sequential motion tasks are increased from two to three different syllables, performance would be expected to deteriorate. Speech production would not be expected to reveal significant motoric struggle; however, movement breakdowns would be expected during longer utterances. This implies more speech errors as utterance length increases. Planning children would be expected to be more verbal than their executive counterparts; yet it would be unlikely to find a normal degree of expressive language performance if for no other reason than the severity of the phonological deficit. Because the posterior aspects of the continuum are involved in these cases, some deficit in language comprehension would be expected. Comprehension would be expected to be superior to expression and may be intact in some children, depending on how far posterior the dysfunction extends. As stated previously, children at the extreme posterior end of the motor-language continuum would be expected to demonstrate more global language deficits in the absence of primary motor speech impairments.

Hypotheses and Clinical Reality

A cautionary note is indicated at this point. The categories proposed by the motolinguistic model and the associated clinical predictions are hypothetical. Clinicians may recognize some of the predicted characteristics in one child or another, but reality dictates that pure forms are seen infrequently. The motolinguistic model dictates a continuum rather than discrete categories. Also, the focus of the model is motor and speech function, not language function. Given the wide variation often observed among any group of developmental disorders, it is probable that children with executive dysfunction or dysarthria would demonstrate concomitant language comprehension deficits. It is also probable that children may show a mix of both executive and planning deficits. As will be seen in the chapters on evaluation and treatment, this model is intended as a clinical guide based on patterns of functional impairment. It should not be taken as a guideline for labeling children with suspected motor speech disorders. Many issues are inherent in the terms used to classify speech disorders. Some of these issues are addressed in the next section.

Working Definitions

Various terms have been used to describe speech disorders in children. Some seem to follow a specific theoretical orientation; others seem simply to reflect clinical observations. Still others seem to implicate etiologies and/or underlying mechanisms. The historical review in Chapter 1 contained three terms relative to children's disorders of speech production: dysarthria, dyslalia, and dyspraxia (herein not distinguished from apraxia). Additional terms that have been applied to speech disorders in children include functional articulation disorders and phonological disorders. This section offers working definitions of these terms. Working definitions, as applied here, are pragmatic efforts to provide a definition for a commonly used term that may have clinical utility. Although theoretical constructs have been considered relevant to each term, more importance has been attributed to the clinical utility of the term. In this regard, some of the discussion or definitions applied to various terms may be more encompassing than specific theories would allow.

Phonological Disorder

This term makes a good starting point since, at this time, it is commonly applied to many children demonstrating disorders of speech production. Some authors advocate a broad application of the term "phonological" as it applies to children with speech production disorders (Edwards & Shriberg, 1983; Locke, 1983). However, the term "phonology" or "phonological system" more traditionally refers to an organizational system of rules that allows speakers to combine sounds of a language in a meaningful manner. These meaningful sounds of language are termed phonemes (at least in English and similar languages) and are considered abstract, mental phenomena (e.g., Ladefoged, 1975; Liles, 1975). Phonemes are felt to have little direct application to the production of speech. For example, extensive variability in production (i.e., dialect variation or disordered speech) may result in the perception of the same phoneme. From the converse perspective, the manner in which linguistic or mental units become motor activities is a lingering problem for speech researchers (Folkins & Bleile, 1990).

Use of the term phonological disorder typically implies a degree of disorganization within the rule system used to organize phonemes. However, it is possible that there are children who demonstrate speech errors without disorganization in the underlying rule system. Also, there may be children who are able to speak adequately but demonstrate disorganization in the underlying phonological system relative to other language tasks. Therefore, although the term phonological disorder may be used to describe many children with disordered speech production, it does not necessarily imply a deficit in the underlying linguistic organization of the sound system. In other words, the term phonological disorder does not necessarily mean a disordered phonological system from a more traditional, linguistic perspective. Rather, the term phonological disorder has been applied clinically as a descriptor for a variety of speech production deficits. Although this use of the term might serve to place a clinical focus on a particular communicative disorder, it does little to focus attention on potential defective processes underlying the overt speech disorder. Folkins and Bleile (1990) question using the term phonology (specifically, "clinical phonology") to apply to all disorders of speech production. They prefer to conceptually separate linguistic processes of "message construction" from motor processes of speech production.

Functional Articulation Disorder

Aram (1980) posed the question: "Whatever happened to functional articulation disorders?" The focus of her question was the identification of children demonstrating apraxia of speech, dysarthria, or phonological disorder—each considered a subset of articulation disorders. Although the term phonological disorder has dominated as a descriptive label for children with speech production deficits, Aram's rhetorical question focused on key arguments over nomenclature that abounded in the 1970s and early 1980s.

One of the focal arguments surrounding various labels was the nature and consistency of speech production errors. A consistent deficit in production of a sound in many environments (here meaning different sound combinations) may indicate inappropriate articulatory movements. Variation in sound production across environments may indicate poor phonological patterning as the articulatory movements and resulting sound production are appropriate in one context but not in another. Such distinctions have been used to contrast articulation and phonological disorders (Shelton & McReynolds, 1979; Shriberg & Kwiatkowski, 1988). This distinction seems to parallel a concern over division of speech production errors into those that are motorically versus linguistically based (e.g., Folkins & Bleile, 1990). Shelton and McReynolds (1979) used the term "disordered articulation" to refer to inability to produce sounds and in reference to disordered phonological organization. As indicated in preceding discussion, the more recent trend has been to describe these errors collectively as phonological disorders. Whichever term is used, it must be recognized that different processes may be disrupted in speech production, leading to potentially different patterns of speech performance.

Dyslalia

Morley (Morley et al., 1954, 1955) used the term "dyslalia" to refer to transient defects of consonant substitution and omission. The general impression of dyslalia as a mild, transient form of speech disorder remains even though the term is used infrequently at this time. When dyslalia is used in current literature, it seems to apply contrastively to associate or dissociate another variable influencing speech. For example, Brown (1985) mentions that tongue-tie was once thought to be a cause of dyslalia. (He rightly points out that the role of tongue-tie in speech disorders has been overemphasized.) He refers to dyslalia as "the common specific developmental slow speech syndrome" (p. 173). Dyslalia may be considered a subcategory of either phonological disorders or functional articulation disorders, depending on the viewpoint of the user. Brown comments that (as a neurologist) he finds it appealing to consider dyslalia as a mild form of apraxia of speech rather than a separate clinical entity. This is an interesting position that has argumentative potential from a theoretical perspective. In practice, clinicians frequently encounter children who achieve normal "developmental milestones" in most areas, including speech onset, but who seem to be progressing in speech development a little slower than expected. Whether we refer to these children as dyslalic or by some other term, the overall prognosis for improvement without therapy is very good.

Dysarthria

Yorkston, Beukelman, and Bell (1988) point out that the term dysarthria comes from the Greek *dys* + *arthroun* meaning "inability to utter distinctly." Given this origin, it should come as no surprise that Morley and her contemporaries considered speech deficits secondary to anatomic abnormalities in the vocal tract as dysarthrias. In recent literature, however, especially in the field of speech-language pathology, dysarthria has been associated with various neuromotor conditions that impair functions of the vocal tract. In fact, Yorkston and her colleagues (1988) define dysarthria as "a neurogenic motor speech impairment which is characterized by slow, weak, imprecise, and/or uncoordinated movements of the speech mechanism" (p. 2). Dysarthrias have been categorized according to the nature of underlying motor impairment causing the speech disorder (see, for example, Darley, Aronson, & Brown, 1975). Lower motor neuron deficits leading to flaccid paralysis in the speech musculature contribute to flaccid dysarthria. Conversely, upper motor neuron deficits causing spasticity are viewed as the underlying problem in spastic dysarthria. This pattern of classification has become popular, and in general, the pattern of motor impairment and motor speech impairment will be parallel. That is, the speech characteristics will reflect the underlying motor deficit.

The term "cortical dysarthria" may lead to substantial confusion. The hearer of this term must decipher whether the speaker is referring to a form of pseudobulbar palsy, such as the dysarthria described by Worster-Drought as congenital suprabulbar paresis, or some other implied motor speech deficit. Brown (1985) indicates that the term cortical dysarthria has been used synonymously with many other terms—apraxia of speech, aphemia, and phonetic disintegration, to name a few. These terms all relate to disrupted motor speech processes, presumably at the cortical level. The term cortical dysarthria might be viewed as representing a point on a continuum of motor speech deficits. However, without additional specification of the intent of the speaker or the characteristics of the subjects, the term cortical dysarthria probably serves more as a stimulant to aggressive conversation than as a clarifier of a clinical problem.

Apraxia of Speech

Apraxia of speech also is viewed as a motor speech disorder. Recall from Chapter 1 that Morley's terms "dyspraxic dysarthria" and "articulatory dyspraxia" resulted from her attempts to classify various types of dysarthria seen in children (Morley et al., 1954). Pertaining to adult patients demonstrating motor speech impairment after brain damage, Wertz (1985, after Darley, 1969) characterized apraxia of speech as an articulatory disorder resulting from impairment of the capacity to program the positioning of speech muscles and the sequencing of muscle movements for the volitional production of phonemes. He went on in his definition to point out that direct sensorimotor pathology cannot account for the speech deficit (i.e., it is not a dysarthria). This definition is not too distant from the description offered by Morley et al. in 1954 of articulatory dyspraxia pertaining to children: "Movements of the lips, tongue, and palate appeared normal on voluntary movements carried out at the examiner's request, but clumsy and awkward when the children attempted the more complex and rapid movements of articulation" (p. 9). The term gives the impression that individuals demonstrating apraxia of speech will reveal deficient motor activity during speech in the absence of explanatory paralysis/paresis. This seems to be the basic concept of apraxia of speech; however, as reviewed in Chapter 1, the picture is not at all that clear. Many investigators and authors have described, defined, or otherwise portrayed different clinical variants of the disorder termed apraxia of speech. As implied by the preceding motolinguistic model, there may be different patterns of motor and motor speech deficits that may pertain to the concept of apraxia. From both a pragmatic, clinical perspective and a theoretical perspective, it would seem naive to put forth only one apraxia of speech and try to explain the variability demonstrated by individuals thus labeled. A different approach might be to postulate different forms of apraxias of speech in which motor and speech performances demonstrate parallel deficits. From this view, the following definition of *developmental apraxias of speech* is offered.

> **Developmental Apraxias of Speech are a group of phonological disorders resulting from disruption of central sensorimotor processes that interfere with motor learning for speech.**

Because these motor speech disorders should be differentiated from dysar-thrias, the following might be appended:

Paralysis or weakness might be present, but is not sufficient to account for the nature and severity of the observed speech disorder.

By specifying that apraxias are a group of disorders, this definition impli-cates more than one clinical variant. Use of the term phonological disorder implicates a disruption in the developmental organization of the linguistic sound system (phonological system). The presumed etiology of these disor-ders is disrupted central sensorimotor processing relative to speech develop-ment. These disrupted processes are thought to interfere not only with the production of speech at any point in time, but with motor learning for new speech patterns.

The theoretical bases for this position were presented in Chapter 2 and in the first part of this chapter. This definition addresses several issues, but ques-tions remain. A closer look at some of the implications and avoidances of this definition is warranted.

A Group of Disorders—The Apraxias

The motolinguistic model proposed in this chapter forms the basis for identi-fying a *group* of disorders as developmental apraxias of speech. Speech aprax-ias are considered to occur when defective motor/language processes overlap. Different patterns of motor and speech performances have been demonstrat-ed which collectively would fall under the domain of apraxic impairment.

Phonological Disorders?

Identifying speech apraxias as phonological disorders rather than motor speech or articulation disorders reflects the perspective that these children demon-strate disordered organization of the portion of the phonological system that is used for speech production. It is conceivable that the phonological system has functional components used for different aspects of information proc-esses. For example, an "input phonology" may be required to analyze audi-tory input, an "internal phonology" for non-modality-specific functions such as rhyming or phoneme-grapheme transformation, and an "output or pro-duction phonology" used to organize phonemes for speech production. The present definition is superficial in that it addresses only the third of these possibilities. However, consistent with current literature, the term phonolog-ical disorder implicates a disorganization in speech processing at some level above the direct motor impairments seen in dysarthria.

Sensorimotor Processes and Speech Learning

The crux of the definition is "disruption of central sensorimotor processes that interfere with motor learning for speech." The fact is that apraxia is a motor performance deficit. If the term apraxia of speech is to be appropriate it should be applied to children in whom evidence of nonparalytic motor impairment of speech is identified. The definition implies poor motor speech learning as a factor in the development of a disordered phonological system. This point has not been tested directly; however, Heilman, Schwartz, and Geschwind (1975) have demonstrated that adults with limb apraxia do have difficulty learning limb motor tasks. If apraxia is viewed as defective organization, planning, and/or execution of motor behavior, it would be expected to interfere with normal learning of motor performance—including speech. The end result of this motor-learning deficit perspective is that the child will develop a disorganized production phonology as permitted by the underlying motor deficit. In executive cases little speech output might be observed; in planning cases one would expect a larger, but still deviant, production phonology. With development and the adoption of compensatory strategies (see Chapter 2) changes in both motor performance and speech performance would be expected.

Beyond Motor Performance

The emphasis of the motolinguistic model and the definition of developmental apraxias of speech is on motor performance—speech and nonspeech. However, all motor behavior is truly sensorimotor in that movements have sensory antecedents and consequences. An important question focuses on the role of defective auditory processes in impaired speech-language ability. Unfortunately, only limited research has been completed in this area in reference to developmental motor speech disorders. Tallal and her colleagues (Tallal & Piercy, 1974, 1975; Tallal & Stark, 1976; Tallal, Stark, Kallman, & Mellits, 1980) have identified impairments in auditory acoustic-phonetic analysis by children with language impairments. Relative to motor performance, Ojemann and Mateer (1979) found substantial overlap of cortical areas in tasks of oral movement and phoneme identification in patients studied with the cortical stimulation paradigm. Aram and Horwitz (1983) reported that children with developmental apraxia of speech demonstrated auditory-sequencing deficits. Yoss and Darley (1974a) reported similar deficits in addition to auditory discrimination deficits in children with defective articulation. These investigators used nonspeech motor tasks to separate potential apraxic speakers from the remainder of the articulatory defective children. Auditory discrimination and sequencing performances did not differ between these two groups of speech impaired children. Collectively, these observations suggest that children with speech-language impairment may have accompanying deficits in certain auditory processing functions. These deficits may contribute to the development of a disorganized phonological system from the input perspective. It is conceivable that auditory based deficits are somehow related to defective motor speech processes, especially those in the nonparalytic arena such as apraxia of speech. However, a great deal of additional research will be required to relate these input limitations to various patterns of motor speech impairment. In this respect, although the output oriented model presented in this chapter may be guilty of scientific myopia, it has potential for clinical application based on a multitude of clinical and empirical observations.

Apraxias for Everyone?

A final question stemming from this definition might be, "Do all children with speech production deficits demonstrate developmental apraxias of speech to varying degrees?" There is no simple answer to this question. It is possible that varying degrees of severity in motor impairment may create analogous degrees of speech production deficit. Certainly, clinicians are familiar with varying degrees of speech difficulty among children. The real issue surrounding this question is that of underlying processes rather than severity of speech disorder. It is conceivable that certain children have learned "abnormal" phonological patterns from many influences. Some children may demonstrate deviant lexical retrieval and/or phoneme selection processes, others may select the proper phonemes but sequence them inappropriately prior to coding the linguistic message into motor speech specifications. In short, not all developmental deviations in speech production are expected to relate to poor motor-learning abilities. Given the vast amount that is unknown regarding both normal and abnormal speech processes, it is probably wise to be conservative in the application of labels. Developmental apraxia(s) of speech would seem an appropriate label only for children who demonstrate nonparalytic motor speech deficits. The position expressed in this chapter suggests that, in such children, parallel deficits in motor and speech performances may be identified.

Implications and Considerations

Subtyping is difficult among child populations (Lahey, 1990; Stark & Tallal, 1981). Frequently, a general symptom from a complex array of speech-language deficits becomes the focus of clinical attention. Obvious motoric limitations during speech attempts and perhaps during nonspeech tasks may be used to label children as dysarthric or apraxic without further delineation of the motor deficit or description of how observed motor deficits might relate to speech-language problems demonstrated by the child. The model proposed in this chapter attempts to focus clinical attention on these issues. It is intended as a guide to approaching assessment and intervention of children with suspected developmental motor speech disorders rather than a "road map of how to." The model is presented as a continuum rather than a group of discrete categories of motor speech disorders in an attempt to direct clinicians away from a labeling focus. Several relevant clinical issues need to be addressed prior to applying this or any model to the treatment of children with developmental motor speech disorders.

Speech-language disorders are not neat entities that always fall predictably into a single category. This often presents a diagnostic problem for clinicians in prioritizing clinical symptoms and selecting treatment options. Pertaining to developmental motor speech disorders, there may be substantial overlap among so-called diagnostic categories. Individual children will demonstrate concomitant apraxia and language disorder (and dyslexia). Others will show evidence of both apraxia and dysarthria. Still others will show a global deficit that incorporates deficits in all three aspects. It also is obvious that there are different types of oral motor impairment associated with speech disorders in children. What has been conspicuously absent in literature regarding motor speech disorders in children is attention to the characteristics of the oral motor deficit in reference to speech characteristics. By focusing on patterns of functional impairment rather than on classification via general symptoms, clinicians and researchers may come to a better understanding of developmental motor speech disorders.

The historical review, the neurolinguistic perspective, and the motolinguistic model each indicate multiple aspects that should be considered when undertaking clinical evaluation and treatment of children with developmental motor speech disorders. Some of these might be considered "rule-in" phenomena. That is, certain characteristics would be expected to be seen that would contribute to the identification of a motor speech disorder. Other aspects might be considered "rule-out" phenomena. These are characteristics that would not be expected to contribute to a specific motor speech disorder. Still other aspects might be "first cousins" or "innocent bystanders." These would be characteristics that would not be important in identification of a motor speech disorder, but which are known to co-occur frequently with speech disorders.

The clinical management of children with suspected motor speech disorders must consider basic motor performance abilities of the speech mechanism (as well as general motor abilities), motor speech characteristics, speech-articulation (phonologic) characteristics, language (spoken, written) abilities, and potentially related academic performance, and interactions among these various characteristics. The remaining chapters review studies of the various functions in developmental dysarthria (congenital suprabulbar paresis) and developmental apraxia of speech and describe evaluation and therapy techniques for the various developmental motor speech disorders.

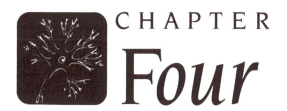

C H A P T E R

Four

Developmental and Clinical Profiles

Someone once said that you never have to convince your friends and you will never be able to convince your enemies. This saying seems appropriate applied to the realm of developmental motor speech disorders, especially developmental apraxias of speech. Writings discussing this topic are replete with controversy and contradiction. The isolated dysarthria seen in congenital suprabulbar paresis seems less controversial; primarily because it has received little attention since the descriptions of Worster-Drought. Yet, from some descriptions of apraxic children, one might wonder if there is confusion between this dysarthria and certain forms of apraxia of speech. Traditionally, apraxia of speech has been presented as a unitary construct focusing on overt motoric struggle and selected characteristics of articulation deficit. Developmental dysarthria, as described by Morley et al. (1954) and Worster-Drought (1974), is depicted as a focal spastic weakness within the speech mechanism that interferes with speech production. Yet, any clinician who has had the opportunity to interact with these children realizes the oversimplification of these positions. Children with developmental motor speech disorders present a complex clinical picture. Because the disorders are present from the earliest developmental stages, there is a strong potential for negative interaction with other developmental skills. Because these disorders tend to result in severe, often persistent, communication problems, there is a clinical motivation to identify children at risk for these disorders at an early age. Yet, despite the clinical importance of these issues, confusion and controversy continue to surround even the most general traits of developmental motor speech disorders. To address this confusion and controversy, this chapter discusses general characteristics that have been attributed to children with developmental motor speech disorders.

Developmental Issues

Two aspects of early development frequently arise in reference to developmental motor speech disorders: developmental milestones and genetic considerations. Do children with motor speech disorders achieve developmental milestones at expected times? Is there a pattern among those milestones which may not be achieved within expected time frames? Recently much attention has been given to potential genetic components of various speech and other learning disorders. Chapter 2 introduced the concept of a possible genetic component in developmental motor speech disorders. Is family history/genetic predisposition an important clinical feature of children with developmental motor speech disorders? Answers to these and other questions may facilitate a better understanding of developmental motor speech disorders and lead to the formulation of a better clinical profile of these children. This step may lead to improved diagnosis and hence better treatment. This perspective launches the following discussion of developmental issues.

Babbling and Speech-Language Development

Worster-Drought (1974) did not delineate general developmental characteristics associated with congenital suprabulbar paresis; however, a rather clear pattern does emerge from his 13 detailed case studies. Of the 13 cases presented, four children were reported to develop normally until confirmed neurologic events (high fevers, convulsions, encephalitis) occurred within the first year of life. Of the remaining nine cases, six children demonstrated late onset of speech attempts with little or no babbling reported prior to speech onset. At onset speech was not considered normal for the child's age. Three children demonstrated expected babbling patterns; however, of these, one did not begin to use meaningful words until 5 years of age, one demonstrated slowed speech acquisition beginning at 14 months, and one demonstrated a dysarthria characterized by hypernasality beginning with emergence of first words. Thus, a relatively high percentage of children later diagnosed as presenting congenital suprabulbar paresis demonstrated little or no babbling and a delay in the emergence of first meaningful words. When first words did emerge, they were felt to be poorly articulated even considering the child's age.

Referencing developmental apraxia of speech, Morley (1965) felt that 4 of the 12 children she studied demonstrated delayed onset of single words and 5 demonstrated delayed emergence of phrases. She offered no commentary on early babbling. Rosenbek and Wertz (1972) felt that all of their 50 apraxic subjects demonstrated delayed onset of speech. However, only 18% of their group was considered to demonstrate an isolated speech disorder, and children with mental retardation were included in their study. Aram and Glasson (1979) claimed to have studied a relatively isolated apraxia of speech in eight children. Four of these children were described as quiet babies who did not babble, and all demonstrated a delay in the emergence of single words and phrases. Average age for emergence of first words was 2.9 years, and phrases emerged at an average of 4.2 years. This is somewhat later that the developmental pattern reported by Morley who described instances of normal and even early speech development among her 12 cases of developmental apraxia of speech.

An interesting observation not often discussed in reference to speech-language development in these children is the temporal relationship between emergence of single words and phrases. Of 12 children, Morley described one case as "early" in both categories and listed no age for onset of single words for another. Of the remaining 10 cases, 50% (5 of 10) demonstrated emergence of phrases within 6 months of the onset of single words. The remaining 50% demonstrated a lag of just over 2 years between the onset of single words and phrases. Six of the eight cases reported by Aram and Glasson demonstrated emergence of phrases within 1 year of the emergence of single words. A single case demonstrated phrases 1.5 years after single words, and the final case had a lag of 4.5 years. It is difficult to make conclusions from limited samples; however, there would seem to be two possible subgroups in these findings with one group demonstrating a shorter time lag between onset of single words and phrases than the other.

Crary (1984a) also reported a high incidence of delayed speech onset. Of 20 children with developmental apraxia of speech, 17 did not use first words until after 2 years of age. Two additional children were reported to have normal speech development until nearly 2 years of age and then to regress, and one child was reported to begin speaking at the expected time, but later demonstrated speech deficits. Information beyond emergence of first words was available for 10 of these children. From chart review and/or parent interview, presence of early babbling, approximate age of first word emergence, word combination, and complete sentence use was identified. In addition, use of communicative gestures was ascertained. Summarized results from the 10 cases are presented in Table 4–1.

Trends similar to those reported by Morley and Aram and Glasson may be seen in Table 4–1. Single words demonstrated a late emergence as did word combinations and complete sentence use. Four of the children began to use word combinations within 6 months of single word use, and only three children demonstrated a lag of more than 1 year. Similarly, in the four children using complete sentences, the lag between word combinations and sentence use was within a year. Half of the children were reported not to have babbled, and 70% were reported to have used communicative gestures either in

Table 4-1. Summary of early language development characteristics for 10 children with developmental apraxia of speech.

Age (in years)	Babbling	First Words (in years)	Combined Words (in years)	Sentences (in years)	Gestures
3.1	No	3	–	–	Yes
3.2	No	2	2	3	
3.3	No	2	3	–	Yes
3.6	No	2	3	–	Yes
3.6		2	2.6	3	Yes
3.8	No	2.6	3	–	
3.8		2	2.6	–	Yes
4.0		2	3	3.6	
4.1		2	4	–	Yes
4.9		2	4	4.3	Yes

Note: Missing data indicate no available information. "–" indicates performance level not demonstrated at time of evaluation.

replacement for, or in addition to, speech attempts. There seems to be no obvious pattern among absence of babbling, use of gesture, onset of first words, and lag between first words and word combinations.

Because these data were gathered from file review and/or parent interview, appropriate caution should be used in interpretation. However, in agreement with prior reports, these data suggest that children demonstrating developmental apraxia of speech have delayed onset of speech. Furthermore, there seems to be a high incidence of absence of babbling and use of gestures to communicate. Finally, in nearly 50% of children studied, the emergence of single words, word combinations, and/or sentences seems to follow a timely pattern. One must wonder if these developmental patterns are the result of other influences or the manifestation of different types of developmental motor speech disorders—in this case different forms of apraxia of speech.

Motor Development

The dysarthria described by Worster-Drought (1974) as part of the syndrome of congenital suprabulbar paresis was presented as a focal "cerebral palsy of the mouth." In this regard, Worster-Drought did not delineate abnormalities in motor development, excepting those cases presenting "hard" neurological deficits relating to cerebellar or direct motor system impairment and even these were few in number. What Worster-Drought did emphasize was the presence of motor deficits related to corticobulbar impairment. Primary among these was difficulty with feeding from a very early age and, especially in the more severe cases, difficulty controlling saliva. These symptoms typically occur in the presence of identifiable paresis/paralysis within the corticobulbar musculature. However, drooling may not be a differential diagnostic feature of dysarthria. Rosenbek and Wertz (1972) reported that 11 of the 50 apraxic children they reviewed demonstrated excessive drooling, including 6 who demonstrated a focal oral apraxia or generalized apraxia in the absence of paresis/paralysis.

Among children with developmental apraxias of speech, a more widespread motor clumsiness may be seen. When present, the "clumsy child syndrome" may create significant difficulty for a child who already possesses a severe speech-language disorder. Consider the following description from Cermak (1985):

> Although poor gross motor coordination may present as a difficulty with total body balance, ineptness may be even more apparent with complex motor activities. Play skills such as learning to ride a tricycle and bicycle, skipping rope, and catching a ball are often achieved at a later age, and seem to take extra effort. The dyspractic child cannot keep up with his peers in sports. He is often the last to be chosen for the team, or excluded from the activity. Some children prefer to play more sedentary games, to play alone, or to play with younger children. (p. 229)

This is a real-life depiction of a significant motor impairment. Although Cermak is not addressing speech apraxia directly, Gubbay (1978) observed that nearly one third of 5- to 12-year-old children who were "generally dyspractic" had accompanying speech difficulties. Rosenbek and Wertz (1972) reported that one third (12 of 36) of their apraxia of speech subjects demonstrated a generalized apraxia. In fact, generalized "clumsiness" or poor coordination is frequently mentioned in reference to developmental apraxia of speech (Ferry, Hall, & Hicks, 1975; Yoss & Darley, 1974a). Aram and Glasson (1979) reported that six of seven children tested had difficulty on three gross motor tests (standing on one foot, hopping on one foot, and skipping). Three of the seven children had difficulty with coordinated hand tasks. Crary (1984a) reported that 13 of 25 children reviewed had a history of some degree of motor incoordination. For 18 of these 25 children early developmental motor history was available. Factors considered were ability to sit unassisted, stand, walk, and toilet training. Only 3 of the 18 children revealed any delay in achieving the developmental milestones. Two were instances where the child did not walk unassisted until after 18 months of age. However, both of those children were walking by 2 years of age. A single child was considered to be delayed in reaching major motor milestones.

Clearly, *some* children with developmental motor speech disorders will show a general clumsiness; others reveal only a focal, oral motor deficit influencing speech as well as nonspeech functions. Aside from potential feeding-swallowing difficulties associated with oral motor weakness and/or incoordination, early developmental motor milestones seem to be attained at expected times.

Medical Complications

Few studies of developmental motor speech disorders have considered early medical complications as a contributing factor. Worster-Drought (1974) emphasized the "congenital" in congenital suprabulbar paresis and differentiated it from the acquired form in children. Crary (1984a) reported that nearly 50% (12 of 25) of the cases he reviewed revealed a history of significant medical complications within the first 2 years of life with few pre- or perinatal complications. This finding raises suspicion regarding potential post-natal influences and suggests that, rather than having a congenital origin, some cases of developmental motor speech disorders result from early post-natal disruptions to the developing speech-language system.

Genetic Considerations

In describing congenital suprabulbar paresis, Worster-Drought (1974) stated that it is almost certainly the result of a developmental defect of the motor tract and the paresis is present from birth. He noted further that the syndrome was familial in 12 families and present in three pairs of twins. Patton et al. (1986; see Chapter 1) studied one of the families described by Worster-Drought for over three generations. Sufficient familial transmission among males in this family existed to lead these investigators to suggest that some cases of congenital suprabulbar paresis may be inherited as an autosomal dominant trait.

Familial histories are prevalent among children with developmental apraxia of speech. Morley (1965) cited a 50% rate of familial history. Ferry, Hall, and Hicks (1975) noted nearly a 30% rate of family transmission; and Aram and Glasson (1979) reported that five of eight children studied had confirmed family histories of speech, language, and/or learning disorders. Perhaps the most detailed study was reported by Saleeby, Hadjian, Martinkosky, and Swift (1978) who noted that 34 of 66 family members over four generations demonstrated defective speech. Not all of these cases would be considered to present developmental apraxia of speech or dysarthria, but some form of defective speech was present. Saleeby and her colleagues also noted instances in which a family member would have been predicted to have abnormal speech but did not. They attributed this to variation in the expression of the genetic trait. Patton et al. (1986) offered another possibility. They suggested that certain individuals may carry genes for various traits but that these traits may not be expressed unless some pre- or post-natal "trigger" occurs to bring out the trait. Perhaps the medical complications reported by Crary (1984a) serve as adequate triggers for certain types or instances of developmental motor speech disorders.

Do family histories prove genetic transmission? The answer to this question could be a wavering "maybe" or possibly an optimistic "probably" (followed by "in some cases"). Tallal, Townsend, Curtis, and Wulfeck (1991) reported that children with language impairment and positive family histories demonstrated significant differences from language impaired children without family histories. In this respect, the type of speech-language disorder (and its associated characteristics) may be relevant to the genetic transmission issue. Garvey and Mutton (1973) reported sex chromosome abnormalities in three of nine children with normal language comprehension but defective expressive speech. Ratcliffe (1982) reported that 9 of 18 boys with sex chromosome abnormalities demonstrated an apraxic-like speech deficit with normal language comprehension. Such studies raise the issue of sex-linked genetic transmission of certain types of speech-language problems. From this perspective, it is interesting to note that most reports of developmental apraxia of speech indicate a predominance of affected males. Geschwind and Behan (1982) have suggested a genetic link between testosterone, delayed growth in the left hemisphere, developmental learning disorders, and various immune diseases. It will be interesting to see whether future research substantiates this hypothesis. At this time, a valid appraisal would be to state that there is a high incidence of familial trends in developmental motor speech disorders, more males seem to be affected than females, and preliminary genetic information links certain sex chromosome abnormalities to certain types of speech disorders. From a clinical perspective, useful advice was offered by Saleeby and her colleagues (1978):

> If the familial nature of dyspraxia is clearly evident on the pedigree, treatment should be initiated at a very young age. Clinicians will then be able to assume a preventative role, working with these individuals to correct the problem before social and environmental reactions to the disorder severely inhibit the patient's personal growth. (p. 5)

A *Developmental* *Profile*

A Reanalysis

In an attempt to synthesize many of the positions and some of the reported data pertaining to developmental aspects of developmental motor speech disorders, 20 of the cases described in Crary (1984a) have been re-evaluated in more detail. These children were all referred for evaluation based on suspicion of developmental apraxia of speech. At the time of evaluation, they demonstrated a severe articulation/phonological disorder marked by motoric struggle during speech. Each child was of normal intelligence and demonstrated receptive language abilities superior to expressive language abilities. All had normal hearing at the time of contact. The children ranged in age from 3 years 2 months to 4 years 10 months. Seven developmental or contributing factor categories were evaluated: (1) speech-language development exclusive of the articulation deficit, (2) oral mechanism deviations, (3) motor development/deficits, (4) pre- and perinatal factors, (5) post-natal medical complications, (6) psychosocial factors (primarily adjustment issues), and (7) hearing history. These categories were evaluated using a three-point scale: (1) within normal expectations, (2) mild-moderate deviation, and (3) severe deviation. In addition, the presence (+) or absence (−) of early babbling and use of communicative gestures was noted. The results of this reanalysis are presented in Table 4–2. Missing data indicate no information was available for that child in the respective category.

Speech-Language Development

Information on speech-language development was available for 17 of the 20 children. Of these, 15 (88%) were judged to have severe deviations in speech-language development, and none were considered to have demonstrated development within normal expectations. The most common finding was late emergence of first words (>2 years). Frequently, articulation deficits were noted from the onset of speech.

Oral Motor Deficits

Only 13 of the 20 children considered to demonstrate some form of developmental motor speech disorder had information available regarding oral motor deficits. Of these, 10 children were considered to present mild-moderate deficits, primarily incoordination or oral apraxia. Two children were noted to drool inappropriately, but no child had evidence of paralysis within the speech mechanism. No confirmed instances of feeding/swallowing difficulties were found.

Motor Development

Notations on motor development were included for all 20 children. Forty percent (8 of 20) of the cases were considered to demonstrate some deviation in motor performance. For the most part, these deviations represented fine motor incoordination, references to clumsiness, and/or slight delays in attaining motor developmental milestones. One child was consider to have been significantly delayed in reaching major motor developmental milestones.

Pre- and Perinatal Factors

Only 3 of 19 children demonstrated any pre- or perinatal difficulties and 2 of the 3 were twins. In this case prenatal difficulties contributed to premature delivery and low birthweight. Yet, neither twin required prolonged hospitalization. Little is known about the third child with a deviant score in this cate-

Table 4–2. Developmental history summary of 20 children with developmental apraxias of speech.

Speech-Language	Oral	Motor	Pre- or Perinatal	Medical	Psychosocial	Hearing	Babbling	Gestures
3	1	1	1	3	2	1	No	No
3	2	1	1	2	2	2	No	Yes
2	2	2	1	2	2	2		
	2	2	1	3	1	2		Yes
3	1	1	1	1	2	1	No	Yes
3	1	1	1	1	2			Yes
3	1	1	1	3	1	1	Yes	Yes
3		2	1	3	2	1	No	No
3	2	2	2	2		2		Yes
3		1	1	3	1	1		Yes
3		1	1	2	2	1	Yes	No
2	2	1	1	3	1	1	No	No
3	2	2	2	3	1	2	No	Yes
3	2	2	3	3	2	1	No	Yes
		1	1	1		1		Yes
3		1	1	1	2	2		Yes
3		1		2	2	2		Yes
3	2	3		1	2	2	No	
3	2	1	1	1	1	2		Yes
3	2	2	1	2	2	1	No	Yes

Note: 1 = within normal expectations, 2 = mild-moderate deviation, 3 = severe deviation. Missing data indicate no available information for that category.

gory because he was adopted. The score in this category is based on the report that his natural mother overdosed on phenobarbital during the pregnancy.

Post-Natal Medical Factors

Post-natal medical factors were frequent in this group. Seventy percent (12 of 20) of these cases were judged to have some deviation in this category. Half of these were considered mild to moderate deviations not requiring hospitalization, including chronic colds, upper respiratory infections, and/or allergies. Severe deviations were noted if hospitalization was required. Many of these instances were associated with seizure activity (secondary to high fevers or reactions to medications) or severe respiratory infections.

Hearing

All children had normal hearing at the time of contact. However, just under 50% of the cases (9 of 19) were considered to demonstrate some degree of hearing difficulty during early development. This proportion may be somewhat inflated as children with chronic colds or upper respiratory infections were considered at risk for ear problems and received a score of 2 in this category. None of the children had confirmed histories of chronic hearing deficits or otologic difficulties.

Psychosocial Adjustment

Just over 60% of these children (12 of 19) were reported to demonstrate some adjustment difficulties. These were primarily in reaction to communication failure, and none was considered to be a severe problem. The majority of these reports included overt frustration at failed communication marked by outbursts or crying. Other frequent notations included reluctance to speak even to family members and/or general shyness and withdrawal from social situations. Perhaps the most severe cases involved children who vomited when attending speech-language therapy.

Gestures and Babbling

Finally, similar to the information presented in Table 4–1, a high percentage of children used gestures communicatively (77%). Eighty-two percent (9 of 11) of these children were noted not to have babbled during early developmental periods. Many of these were considered to be quiet babies who were "easy to care for."

These observations seem to be in good agreement with many previous, fragmented reports of developmental characteristics of children with developmental motor speech disorders. The pattern seems to be one in which babbling is absent in early development followed by a delay in the emergence of first words, articulation errors present from the onset of speech, and frequent use of communicative gestures. Generalized motor deficits are infrequent and when present are manifested as clumsiness. Major developmental motor milestones typically are reached within expected time frames. Little evidence exists to support abnormal pre- or perinatal conditions as contributing factors, but post-natal medical factors may play a role. These conclusions and trends are not etched in stone. Children were observed who did not match the group trends. Yet, the patterns noted from these 20 children and those reported previously do provide a clinical perspective on developmental issues when a developmental motor speech disorder is suspected.

Clinical Profiles

What do children with developmental motor speech look like? An occupational therapist once commented that she could pick out her "clumsy children" from a crowded waiting room. These were typically boys with disheveled hair, shirts incorrectly buttoned, zippers down, shoes untied, and glasses askew. It would be convenient, if not advantageous, if there was a distinguishing group of characteristics like these that identified children with developmental motor speech disorders. Unfortunately, this is not the case, and the diagnostic profile of children with developmental apraxia of speech has been a highly controversial topic for many years. Perhaps, one reason why the dysarthria associated with congenital suprabulbar paresis has not created a diagnostic dilemma is that this entity has received little attention in speech-language pathology literature. Yet, it is possible that some children demonstrating dysarthria associated with congenital suprabulbar paresis are confused with children demonstrating certain forms (primarily executive) of apraxia of speech. Also, it is probable that there are children who present with both a dysarthria and an apraxia of speech. This mixing of deficits along with the historical lack of recognition of apraxia variants may well be one source of much of the confusion and controversy surrounding developmental motor speech disorders. Another source of confusion seems to be the lack of "purity" involved in developmental motor speech disorders. Many of these children may demonstrate associated language deficits and/or other learning deficits. A third potential source of confusion may be developmental changes in the clinical profile. It is not realistic to expect a 3-year-old child to demonstrate the same characteristics as a 7- or 8-year-old child. In this regard there seem to be two issues to address: (1) What clinical characteristics historically have been attributed to developmental motor speech disorders? and (2) Is there a common core of symptoms that aid in clinical identification of these disorders?

Historical Attributes

Dysarthria

Dysarthria associated with congenital suprabulbar paresis would seem to be easily identifiable. Worster-Drought (1974) indicated that this disorder is characterized by an isolated weakness of musculature innervated by the cranial nerves, primarily motor nerves to the face, tongue, and palate. He further stated that the weakness is of the upper motor neuron variety. Less than 25% of the cases involved the complete syndrome; the remaining cases demonstrated variability of involvement of the lips, tongue, and palate. From a clinical perspective then, a cluster of identifiable symptoms appears to lead to a diagnosis of congenital suprabulbar paresis and the associated dysarthria. An isolated upper motor neuron weakness of the lips, tongue, and/or palate would be expected to create speech and feeding/swallowing problems as a direct result of the weakness. The pattern of speech disturbance would be expected to relate directly to the involved anatomy. Labial weakness would produce difficulty with labial sound production; lingual weakness would produce lingual misarticulations; and palatal weakness would produce hypernasality and possibly deficits in lingua-velar consonants. This clinical profile is in harmony with that presented by Morley and her colleagues (1954) who differentiated developmental dysarthria from both the dysarthria of cerebral palsy and from dyslalia (see Chapters 1 and 3). This historic agreement places a clinical focus on symptoms associated with developmental dysarthria that should facilitate clinical identification. It would be a mistake, however, to assume that each child encountered who demonstrated this isolated dysarthria presented no other speech-language or associated deficits. Morley and colleagues (1955) reported that dysarthria might coexist with developmental aphasia. Despite this cooccurrence, they maintained that the two disorders bore no intrinsic relationship. Following extensive study of these children, Worster-Drought (1974) reported a variety of deficits concomitant with congenital suprabulbar paresis in just over half of the children studied. These are reviewed in more detail in Chapter 1; however, it is applicable to point out at this juncture that the most frequent concomitant deficit was "retarded development of spoken language other than defective articulation." Within this group, the most prevalent subtype was expressive language deficit. He also indicated a wide range of intellectual ability among these children, although more than half had intelligence within the normal range. The primary point here is that there seems to be a cluster of agreed-on characteristics that differentiate developmental dysarthria from other speech-language disorders, but that developmental dysarthria also may coexist with other developmental speech-language disorders as well as with other cognitive, learning deficits.

Apraxia of Speech

Developmental apraxia of speech has not and does not enjoy this apparent degree of clinical clarity. Numerous terms have been applied to, presumably, the same disorder over the years, and a variety of subject descriptors have been used to select children for studies on the topic. One cannot help but wonder what Morley might say about all this confusion. She and her colleagues seemed to be quite clear on the delineation of developmental speech disorders from the early publications in the 1950s through her clinical studies published in text form nearly a decade later: Some children may present an isolated developmental dysarthria, some an articulatory apraxia, and some dyslalia. Tantamount among the differentiating features of these deficits was the movement pattern of the vocal mechanism during speech and nonspeech tasks. The child presenting apraxia of speech would have normal movements of the lips, tongue, and palate except during speech production when clumsy and awkward movements were noted. Morley also differentiated speech production patterns among these three diagnostic categories. Finally, she recognized that other deficits may coexist with dysarthria and apraxia of speech but this rarely occurred in cases of dyslalia. She made it sound so simple that one must question the source of continued controversy.

Confusion, Controversy, or Perspective

From the outset it might be wise to separate issues. Confusion in the identification of clinical characteristics is not the same as disagreement regarding which attributes characterize a given disorder. However, disagreement regarding characteristics can lead to confusion in the identification of a disorder. Is there a common core of identifiable symptoms that might lead clinicians to consider developmental apraxia of speech? Different authors have selected subjects and described developmental apraxia of speech in apparently variant manner. In Chapter 3, developmental apraxias of speech were defined as a group of phonological disorders. This perspective and the associated model predict different performance profiles in the different apraxias. Does this imply that each type of apraxia will have its own distinguishing traits? Yes. But, Chapter 3 also emphasized that the label "apraxia" should be reserved only for children who demonstrate nonparalytic motor speech deficits. This view is more traditional and implies common features across the respective developmental motor speech disorders. To set the stage for further discussion it seems mandatory to consider what others have reported or observed about developmental apraxia of speech. The apparent controversy may owe more to perspective than to confusion.

Rosenbek and Wertz

Most of the early investigations of developmental apraxia of speech followed a motor speech orientation similar to that offered by Morley years before. Rosenbek and Wertz (1972) never offered a definition of developmental apraxia of speech, but they stated that the term emphasizes the motoric aspects of speech production thereby separating this disorder from a more central language impairment. Among the characteristics associated with developmental apraxia of speech, these investigators included: coexistence of aphasia and/or dysarthria, receptive language abilities superior to expressive, frequent occurrence of oral nonverbal apraxia, and groping, trial-and-error movements during speech. They also suggested certain speech performance characteristics that might differentiate apraxia of speech from other types of speech impairment. Some of these characteristics were not specifically addressed by Morley, but there is no indication that these characteristics are in conflict with her perspective of this disorder.

Yoss and Darley

Yoss and Darley (1974a) followed a slightly different path to the identification of characteristics associated with developmental apraxia of speech. These investigators evaluated a group of children with speech articulation deficits and divided them into two subgroups based on performance on an oral motor task. They controlled both intelligence and language performance factors when selecting their subjects. The possibility of dysarthria was limited in their subject group by excluding children who may have demonstrated "organic" disability as the primary cause of the speech disorder. Yoss and Darley concluded that one of their subgroups was appropriately described by the label "developmental apraxia of speech." These children differed from the other subgroup of misarticulating children not only on performance on isolated oral movement tasks, but also on sequential oral movement tasks and on severity of "soft" neurological deficits. Common among these neurologic signs were decreased lingual alternate motion rates and gait and coordination difficulties. Again we see that, although the perspective of this investigation differed from earlier efforts, a common core of clinical signs emerges. Children with developmental apraxia of speech are depicted as having severe speech articulation deficits in combination with signs of volitional oral motor limitations. The specifics may vary, but the theme is constant.

Ferry, Hall and Hicks

Ferry, Hall and Hicks (1975) took an approach similar to Rosenbek and Wertz (1972) in their description of the clinical characteristics of developmental apraxia of speech. Unlike Rosenbek and Wertz, however, these investigators defined the disorder and stated the criteria used for subject selection. They defined this disorder as

> a neurological disorder of speech manifest by impaired ability—in the absence of overt motor or sensory paralysis—to carry out purposeful movements of the organs of articulation." (1975, p. 719)

By this definition they have limited the possibility of including dysarthric children in their group. Their selection criteria included: (1) delay in speech onset, (2) normal hearing, (3) receptive language normal or superior to expressive, (4) inconsistent speech articulation errors, (5) more articulation errors on more complex phonetic combinations, (6) groping and struggle of the oral articulators, (7) an elaborate gesture system, and (8) limited progress in speech therapy. The results of this study were similar in many respects to prior descriptions of children with developmental apraxia of speech. A high incidence of oral motor problems (orofacial apraxia) was identified (over one half of the cases) as was the presence of nonoral motor deficits (over one third of the cases). These authors are among the few who have indicated a "nearness" of developmental apraxia of speech to the dysarthria seen in congenital suprabulbar paresis. They suggest that there are many overlapping features in the disorders and that the distinctions between them may be more of degree than of difference. However, given the inclusion of retarded individuals in their study and the reported severity of some of the oral "vegetative" deficits, the possibility that some of these individuals presented an undetected dysarthria, either concomitant with the apraxia of speech or in isolation, must be considered.

Aram

Each of these reports emphasized the motoric aspects of developmental apraxia of speech. Aram (Aram & Glasson, 1979; Aram & Nation, 1982) took a slightly different perspective toward developmental *verbal* apraxia. Although she recognized and agreed with the motor speech component of this disorder delineated by previous investigators, she felt that the selective emphasis on speech production did not adequately reflect the extent of disruption to the developing speech-language system. To demonstrate this disruption, Aram and Glasson (1979) and later Ekelman and Aram (1983, 1984) provided detailed analysis of receptive and expressive language abilities. Consistent with prior perspectives, she reported that receptive language functions were superior to expressive functions. However, she noted that increased length of input seemed to have a negative influence on comprehension. Expressive language deficits were prominent; primarily in reference to syntactic formulation, but semantic formulation deficits also were noted. Aram also supported the perspective that some of these children demonstrated more widespread learning disabilities, specifically in reference to reading, writing, and spelling. Although many of Aram's observations agreed with prior reports of associated deficits in apraxia of speech, her perspective differed. Rather than viewing these deficits as concomitant, Aram felt that the observed language deficits were an integral part of this developmental motor speech disorder.

Crary

In a series of studies Crary (1984a, 1984b; Crary, Landess, & Towne, 1984; Crary & Towne, 1984) utilized a strategy similar to Aram's and focused on a "core clinical profile" in selecting subjects to address questions about developmental apraxia of speech. The primary attribute of his subjects was multiple speech articulation errors in the presence of observed "motoric incoordination" during speech tasks. No subject demonstrated obvious evidence of direct sensorimotor pathology in the speech mechanism that would contribute to dysarthria. All subjects had language comprehension abilities within the normal range on standardized tests. Expressive language abilities were variable but typically inferior to receptive abilities. Each child demonstrated intelligence within the normal range either by standardized testing or by academic performance. Hearing was within normal limits, and children with histories of chronic otitis media were not included among his observations. Crary's position was somewhere between the traditional view and Aram's perspective. He emphasized the motor speech component of developmental apraxia of speech, but he espoused a "phonological disorganization" point of view. Also, although he agreed with Aram's observations of deficit syntactic expression, he felt that these limitations were secondary to the primary disruption in the developing phonological system.

A Core of Clinical Characteristics: Is There a Common Ground?

The perspectives of the more recent investigators do not disagree with the traditional view of developmental apraxia of speech as a developmental motor speech disorder. Rather, they expand the range of potential deficits that may coexist with or be inherent to various types of developmental motor speech disorders. The common ground among these positions is a severe deficit in speech articulation ability accompanied by overt signs of motor difficulty during speech. A concomitant nonspeech oral apraxia is frequently, but not always, present. Likewise, an expressive language deficit is frequently noted. This is consistent with the initial writings of Morley. Yet, each of these studies chose subjects differently and described different aspects of this developmental motor speech disorder. Despite these differences, there seems to be a common core of characteristics associated with developmental apraxia of speech. Reported differences seem to be related to the perspective of the various authors rather than to confusion/controversy regarding the nature of developmental apraxia of speech. Table 4–3 summarizes some of the more salient nonspeech characteristics that have been associated with developmental apraxia of speech and congenital suprabulbar paresis. Collectively, these observations represent over 130 children with developmental apraxia of speech in addition to the 200 dysarthric children studied by Worster-Drought.

Genetic Predisposition

Investigators who have questioned the potential for genetic predisposition among children with developmental motor speech disorders have concluded that there is a strong possibility for genetic transmission. The evidence in support of this position varies widely, frequently relying on observations of fa-

Table 4–3. Summary of general clinical features historically associated with developmental motor speech disorders.

Characteristic	Report						
	Morley (1965)	Rosenbek & Wertz (1972)	Yoss & Darley (1974a)	Ferry, Hall, & Hicks (1975)	Aram & Glasson (1979)	Crary (1984a)	Worster-Drought (1974)
Genetic predisposition	+			+	+	+	+
Abnormal speech-language development	+/−	+		+	+	+	+/−
Receptive > Expressive		+		+	+	+	+/−
Abnormal motor development/function		+	+/−	+	+/−	+/−	
Oral apraxia	+/−	+	+	+	+	+	
Normal intelligence		+/−	+	+/−	+	+	+

Note: + = characteristic frequently associated, +/− = characteristic noted less than 50% occurrence. Missing data indicate "characteristic not addressed."

milial trends. The information presented earlier in this chapter and the recent increased emphasis on genetic aspects of communicative disorders in general point to an expanding and exciting area of future investigation in developmental motor speech disorders.

Speech-Language Development

Morley was the only investigator who did not feel that apraxic children, as a group, demonstrated deviant speech-language development. She did describe instances of delayed onset of words and/or phrases; however, she also reported cases of normal language development. The remaining investigators, except Yoss and Darley who did not address this issue, reported that most apraxic children demonstrated abnormal patterns of speech-language development. Worster-Drought's reports of dysarthric children leave the door open for varying interpretations. Of the 200 children studied, slightly more than 25% demonstrated language problems. These children would be considered to present deviant speech-language developmental patterns. Worster-Drought did not specially address developmental milestones among his reported statistics. Yet, in his case reports, there is a high incidence of deviant speech-language development beyond abnormal speech production. In this regard and with consideration of the congenital nature of the dysarthria described by Worster-Drought, it is highly probable that there is a high incidence of deviant speech-language development among children with congenital suprabulbar paresis.

Language Abilities

A similar pattern is noted for perceptions of the general language profile of children with developmental motor speech disorders across the respective reports. Morley specified a concomitant developmental aphasia in some of the children she observed. Unfortunately, there was no detailed reference to the pattern of language performance. Yoss and Darley's subject selection criteria precluded interpretation of receptive-expressive language functions, although overall language performance of their subjects was within normal expectations. With the exception of Rosenbek and Wertz, the remaining investigators chose their apraxic subjects based, in part, on a receptive-expressive language split. Thus, the Rosenbek and Wertz report stands as the least biased indicator and supports the general perspective of superior receptive language abilities among children with developmental apraxia of speech. Dysarthric children may present a slightly different picture. When all 200 children were considered, the incidence of language deficits was low. However, when language deficits were observed, the dominant pattern was receptive language abilities superior to expressive. In general, if a child with a developmental motor speech disorder reveals deficits in language abilities, one would expect an imbalance in language performance favoring receptive functions. Clinicians should be advised that this observation may be dependent on other factors such as nonverbal intelligence (Aram & Nation, 1982).

Motor Milestones

Limited information is available concerning motor development and the presence of motor deficits. Both Rosenbek and Wertz and Ferry, Hall, and Hicks reported a relatively high percentage of "hard" motor signs (paresis, spasticity, hyperkinesia) among their apraxic subjects. However, both of these reports included individuals with mental retardation, adding potential bias to their observations. The remaining three apraxia reports addressing this issue (Morley did not) implicate the presence of generalized motor incoordination among apraxic children. It is difficult to form conclusions from these observations, however, because the reports varied widely in the procedures used to identify motor limitations. Likewise, there is limited information on motor development in these children. Crary (Table 4-2) suggests that apraxic children generally do not demonstrate significant delays in reaching major motor milestones. Other reports barely address this issue among children with apraxia of speech. Children with congenital suprabulbar paresis are not expected, by definition, to demonstrate more generalized motor deficits. Worster-Drought emphasized the focal, corticobulbar nature of this disorder. The tentative conclusion is that children with developmental motor speech disorders do not demonstrate significant gross motor developmental deviations. However, some may demonstrate a degree of generalized motor incoordination. There is simply too little systematic information to reach any conclusion regarding the incidence, extent, and severity of general motor limitations among these children.

Nonspeech Oral Motor Deficits

The presence of nonspeech, oral motor control deficits is considered separately from generalized motor performance issues. With the exception of Rosenbek and Wertz and Ferry, Hall, and Hicks, there is little mention of vegetative deficits within the oral mechanism (drooling, feeding, and swallowing problems) among apraxic children. Conversely, all of these reports noted the presence of oral apraxia. Although Morley did not address this finding beyond noting that it may accompany the speech disorder, each of the other reports emphasized difficulty with nonspeech volitional oral movement. Worster-Drought offered no description of potential oral apraxia among dysarthric children. Apparently, oral apraxia is considered a dominant, although not mandatory, attribute of development apraxia of speech. The relation of oral apraxia to developmental dysarthria is poorly delineated.

Intelligence

In most cases of developmental motor speech disorders, intelligence is reported to be within a normal range. There are, however, reported instances of both apraxia of speech and dysarthria among individuals with below normal intelligence. The underlying deficits in developmental motor speech disorders do not seem related directly to intellectual abilities; yet, there is potential overlap between the two areas.

A General Clinical Profile

The summary in Table 4–3 depicts a general clinical profile of the child demonstrating a developmental motor speech disorder. There is a tendency for familial transmission and abnormal speech-language development beyond the motor speech disorder. Receptive language functions may be expected to be superior to expressive language functions. Motor development seems to follow a timely course, but there may be evidence of generalized motor incoordination. Oral apraxia seems prevalent among children with apraxia of speech but has not been well studied among dysarthric children. These disorders may occur in children along the continuum of intelligence, although many reports of children with developmental motor speech disorders have indicated intelligence within normal limits. This general profile is superimposed on the overt presence of a severe speech production deficit that reflects motor incoordination during speech attempts.

Multiple Forms

Investigators traditionally have ignored the possibility that different forms of speech apraxias may exist. This traditional emphasis on a unitary form of developmental apraxia of speech, stated or implied, contributes further to the controversy and confusion surrounding developmental motor speech disorders. The motolinguistic model directly addresses this issue and contends that motor and speech performances may be envisioned along a continuum from purely motor speech difficulties (i.e., dysarthria) to purely central language difficulties (i.e., specific language impairment). The point is that developmental motor speech disorders *are* a variable group of clinical entities. The common denominator among these variants is the coexistence and presumed interrelationship of speech articulation and motor performance deficits. These deficits may well have an influence on the overall development of the child's language system—especially expressive aspects of language. A single label is simply inadequate to communicate all of the intricacies of the observed performances or the relationships among motor, speech, and language functions. It is unlikely that perfect agreement will ever be reached on clinical nomenclature. Rather than arguing over appropriate labels for observed characteristics, a more positive clinical approach would be to develop strategies for the evaluation of motor, speech, and language abilities and their potential interactions. This process-oriented approach may serve well in the clinical evaluation of any child with a speech-language disorder, but it should be given primary consideration whenever a developmental motor speech disorder is suspected. The ensuing chapters review motor, speech, and language characteristics of children with developmental motor speech disorders in more detail. Wherever possible, the reported signs and symptoms in each of these areas will be related to the motolinguistic model presented in Chapter 3.

Think About This

There is substantial and heated controversy focusing on the specific characteristics of children with developmental motor speech disorders. Still, a common core of attributes is perpetuated across the various perspectives. These include:

1. A tendency for familial transmission of speech-language and/or learning disorders.
2. Delayed onset of speech and deviant speech-language development.
3. Variability in receptive language abilities but typically superior receptive compared to expressive abilities.
4. Major motor milestones are achieved in timely fashion but there may be signs of generalized incoordination.
5. Observable oral paresis in dysarthric children and a high incidence or oral apraxia among children with apraxia of speech.
6. Clinical characteristics may change over time, possibly related to the child's ability to compensate for deficits.
7. **A severe and persistent speech production deficit that may be present from the emergence of first words.**

These observations may form the core of a general clinical profile depicting children with developmental motor speech disorders. They should not be considered to reflect stringent diagnostic criteria. Substantial variability in observed characteristics is to be expected among children with developmental motor speech disorders because they are a diverse group. The general clinical profile discussed in this chapter is the beginning rather than the end of the trail of clinical investigation.

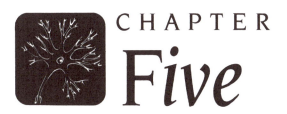

C H A P T E R

Five

Motor Performance

Perhaps the key word in "developmental motor speech disorders" is *motor*. Whether the focus is on dysarthria or on the apraxias, the overt implication is that deviant motor processes contribute directly to the presence and characteristics of these speech disorders. But, what do we really know about the motor functions and/or limitations of children with developmental motor speech disorders? Several issues need consideration in reference to impaired motor performance in children with developmental motor speech disorders. Practical clinical issues include the presence and nature of oral motor impairments, limb motor impairments, motor speech impairments and potential relationships among oral, limb, and motor speech limitations.

In cases of congenital suprabulbar paresis the presence of oral motor and motor speech deficits and their relationship is often overt. These children will present abnormal reflexes associated with corticobulbar deficits. They may present early, severe, and persistent vegetative dysfunctions of oral skills such as sucking, chewing, swallowing, and controlling saliva. Their articulation errors are thought to correlate directly with the anatomy of the upper motor neuron paresis. If lip musculature is paretic, lip sounds will be defective. If velar musculature is paretic, speech will be characteristically hypernasal. There is little concern about limb motor deficits in this disorder because the focus is on the corticobulbar musculature. However, as we change focus to the child with a developmental apraxia of speech, the clarity of motor findings expected in the dysarthric child disappears. Clear neurologic guidelines to identify oral, limb, and motor speech deficits and to evaluate their potential interrelatedness are not available. This ambiguity extends to the dysarthric child when we recognize the possibility for dysarthria and forms of apraxia to overlap. In that respect many of the issues surrounding motor performance in the child with an apraxia of speech also apply to the child with dysarthria. This chapter presents a review of findings on motor performance in children with developmental motor speech disorders. Oral, limb, and motor speech performances are addressed as well as their potential interrelationships.

Oral Motor Performance

Basic Observations

In most instances, children with a developmental motor speech disorder will not demonstrate a severe and obvious paralysis within the speech mechanism. The motor deviations seen in these children typically are more subtle pareses, reflex abnormalities, and/or incoordination on vegetative and/or volitional movements. The most overt motor deviations would be expected in the dysarthric child presenting congenital suprabulbar paresis. These children would be expected to demonstrate spastic paresis and abnormal reflexes secondary to suprabulbar deviations in the corticobulbar tract. Still, unless the weakness is of sufficient severity to be obvious, it may be overlooked or deemed insufficient to contribute to the observed speech difficulty. Also, examining reflexes such as the jaw jerk is often difficult, if not impossible, in a less than cooperative child. The child with an apraxia of speech presents an even greater clinical challenge. Typically, these children present no overt signs of neurological deficit. When present, oral motor limitations often are confined to volitional movements and may vary from one child to the next. Evaluating volitional oral movement performance is not a simple and straightforward procedure. Clinicians must confront their beliefs about deviant motor processes in developmental motor speech disorders and select appropriate examination protocols to evaluate as many aspects of deviant motor processes as possible.

Traditional Examinations for Oral Apraxia: Representative Postures

Many terms have been applied to apraxic deficits observed in the oral musculature including oral apraxia, nonverbal apraxia, and buccofacial apraxia. There seem to be no meaningful distinctions among these terms implicating different pathophysiologies or patterns of performance. Likewise, a variety of tasks have been used to test motor performance in cases of suspected oral apraxia. The more traditional approach has been the use of single posture, representative tasks, for example: "Show me how you kiss a baby" or "Puff out your cheeks." The rationale for this approach comes from studies of adults with aphasia which have indicated that motor speech deficits frequently are accompanied by an oral apraxia as measured by such movement tasks (De Renzi,

Pieczuro, & Vignolo, 1966; LaPointe & Wertz, 1974). A clinical example of this approach is seen in the *Dworkin-Culatta Oral Mechanism Examination* (D-COME) (Dworkin & Culatta, 1980). The subtest of this procedure examining oral apraxia includes six single oral gestures: puffing the cheeks, blowing, lip smacking, lip puckering, tongue wiggling, and whistling. The authors state that "groping for accurate posturing of the lips, cheeks, and tongue during volitional nonspeech tasks, without impairment of automatic or reflexive control of these structures, is suggestive of oral apraxia. These findings frequently coexist with apraxia of speech" (Dworkin & Culatta, 1980, p. 58). Ludwig (1983) used this procedure to delineate symptoms of oral apraxia in a study of phonological behavior in children with apraxia of speech. She compared performances of children with apraxia of speech to normal-speaking children matched to the apraxic group on receptive (same chronological age) or expressive (younger children) language ability. None of the normal-speaking children demonstrated groping behaviors on any of the six movement tasks. Among the apraxic group, two movement tasks were performed with no evidence of groping (blowing and tongue wiggle). The lip smacking and lip pucker tasks produced the greatest difficulty for these children as a group, but even in these tasks only 4 and 5 of the 10 children with apraxia of speech demonstrated overt difficulty.

Ludwig's results are similar to those of earlier studies in that 40% to 50% of children with apraxia of speech demonstrated some signs of oral apraxia as assessed by traditional single posture/movement tasks (Aram & Glasson, 1979; Ferry, Hall, & Hicks, 1975; Rosenbek & Wertz, 1972). An interesting finding from these reports is that children with apraxia of speech did not demonstrate difficulty on all tasks and that some children demonstrated no difficulty on any of the tasks. These observations raise questions regarding the method by which oral apraxia is assessed in children with developmental motor speech disorders. The motolinguistic model suggests that single facial postures or movements alone are not a sufficient assessment of potential oral apraxias. Different praxis impairments will require different assessment strategies. Specifically, consideration should be given to contrasting single postures or movements with the same postures/movements embedded in a sequence.

Single Postures and Movement Sequences

Perhaps the best known study of nonspeech facial movement performance in children with speech articulation deficits was done by Yoss and Darley (1974a). These investigators utilized a modified version of De Renzi, Pieczuro, and Vignolo's (1966) test for oral apraxia. This procedure included 14 single movement facial tasks (show me how you blow, puff out your cheeks, show me how you whistle, etc.) and two- and three-movement sequences (presumably the same tasks used to assess single movements). Yoss and Darley reported that speech-disordered children performed poorer than normal-speaking children on these tasks. They also identified two apparent subgroups among the children with speech disorders. The two subgroups were differentiated on the basis of performance on single movement facial tasks. Both groups were equally impaired on performance of sequential movement tasks. Yoss and Darley suggested that the subgroup of children with poor single movement performance might be appropriately described by the label developmental apraxia of speech. Even though the speech-disordered children who performed better on the single movement tasks performed poorer than the normal-speaking children on the sequential movement tasks, Yoss and Darley did not consider them to represent a motor speech deficit that would qualify as an apraxia of speech. The motolinguistic model might consider both groups of speech-impaired children to reflect an apraxia of speech. The subgroup demonstrating poor performance on both single and sequential movements might be considered to present an executive form of apraxia, whereas the children performing poorly only on the sequential tasks might present a planning variant of apraxia.

Aram and Horwitz (1983) used the test of volitional oral movements outlined by Spriestersbach, Morris, and Darley (1978) as their assessment of "nonspeech oral praxic abilities." This procedure is similar to that used by Yoss and Darley (1974a) in that various single movements are evaluated followed by performance of some of these movements in two- and three-movement sequences. Aram and Horwitz (1983) reported that only 40% of their group of children demonstrating apraxia of speech had difficulty with single oral movement tasks, but 80% of these children had difficulty with sequential oral movements. Dewey, Roy, Square-Storer, and Hayden (1988) felt that performance of single oral movements was not useful in differentiating dyspraxic from nondyspraxic children with defective articulation. Movement sequences were considered more discriminating between the two subgroups. These authors felt that reduced performance of sequential tasks was most pronounced on tasks requiring different movements as the children demonstrated difficulty making transitions from one movement to the next.

These three studies differ in their interpretation of impaired motor performance in children with developmental motor speech disorders, specifically developmental apraxia of speech. The crux of the issue appears to be the comparative performance of such children on single movement tasks versus sequential movement tasks. There seem to be children who perform poorly on both single and sequential tasks. In contrast, there seem to be children who perform single movement tasks at the level of normal-speaking children or at least superiorly to their performance on sequential tasks. The motolinguistic model depicts these motor performance differences as different types of apraxias of speech.

Sequencing Deficit or Performance Load Deficit?

Crary and Towne (1984) reported that six children with developmental apraxia of speech had little difficulty with single oral postures but that their performances deteriorated when the same postures were incorporated into movement sequences. No attempt was made to differentiate types of apraxic impairment or to evaluate the characteristics of the motor impairment. The authors concluded that increased sequential complexity of a task contributed to decreased motor performance. Crary and Anderson (1990) evaluated various motor performance indices in children with a developmental apraxia of speech versus normal-speaking control subjects. To evaluate oral motor performance they utilized the facial mimicry tasks developed by Mateer (Mateer, 1978; Mateer & Kimura, 1977; Ojemann & Mateer, 1979). These tasks require the subject to perform nonrepresentational facial postures either in isolation or in a sequence. The facial postures are nonrepresentational in that they have no overt meaning. They included: protrude the lips, lateralize the tongue, elevate the tongue outside of the mouth, open the mouth, protrude the tongue, and bite the lower lip. The procedure requires the subject to produce the isolated facial posture, the same posture three times in a sequence, two different postures in a sequence, and three different postures in a sequence. As shown in Figure 5–1, the performance of the apraxic group deteriorated significantly as the sequential complexity of the movement task increased. Normal-speaking children performed better than children with an apraxia of speech, and their performance was not adversely influenced by sequential complexity level.

These results might be interpreted to indicate that the children with an apraxia of speech had a sequencing deficit because they made more errors on longer sequences. However, analysis of error types did not support this position. Table 5–1 presents the hierarchy of error types observed for this task in the respective groups. The data, representing the tally of occurrences of each error type, indicate that errors of sequence (sequential order) were infrequent. By far the most frequent error was "groping." Groping was defined as trial-and-error movements of the lips, tongue, and jaw during task performance. Groping was most often noted at the initial attempt to execute a movement and between postures in a sequence. Thus, these results do not support a sequencing deficit per se in these children. Rather, they indicate a "performance load deficit." As the performance load was increased by adding new elements to the motor task, performance decreased even though the same movements were used at all levels of complexity.

Implications from the Motolinguistic Model: Performance Profiles

In a further analysis of these data, Crary (1991) considered the evidence for subgroups of apraxic impairment. Specifically, evidence was sought that would support or refute the motolinguistic model. Figure 5–2 depicts the performance predicted by the model for children considered to demonstrate an executive versus a planning form of apraxia. The executive form would be characterized by poor performance on isolated movement tasks with performance

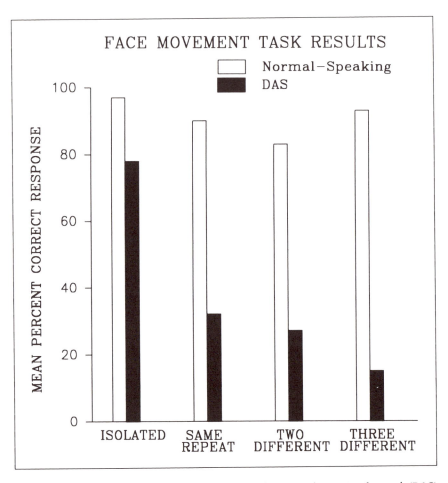

Figure 5–1 Performance of 10 children with developmental apraxia of speech (DAS) compared to 10 normal-speaking children of the same age on the task of volitional nonspeech facial movements. (Data from Crary & Anderson, 1990)

deteriorating as task complexity increased. The planning form would be characterized by a higher level (or normal) performance on isolated tasks with a systematic deterioration in performance in conjunction with increased sequential complexity. Figure 5–3 presents results from three children with apraxia of speech on the oral movement task. The child designated as "executive" is considered to present an executive profile across complexity levels. The children designated "Plan1" and "Plan2" are considered to present planning profiles. Their performance is superior to the executive case at all complexity levels; however, they reveal the predicted decay in performance as sequential complexity increases. Despite the slight increase in performance by Plan2 at the highest complexity level, his overall performance profile is consistent with the "planning deficit profile" predicted by the model.

***Table* 5–1.** Hierarchy of error types for children with apraxia of speech and normal-speaking controls on a nonspeech facial movement task. Ranking is from most to least frequent error type.

Ranking	Apraxic Group	Control Group
1	Groping	Groping
2	Partial response	Incomplete posture
3	Slow release	Slow release
4	Incomplete posture	Partial response
5	Slow initiation	Perseveration
6	Use of hand	Incorrect sequence
7	Incorrect sequence	
8	Added posture (unrelated)	
9	Slow transition	
10	Perseveration	
11	Exaggerated response	
11 (tie)	Vocalization	

Source: Data from Crary and Anderson (1990)

Clinical Considerations

Clinicians must address, or better yet confront, some basic issues regarding oral motor performance in children with overt or suspected developmental motor speech disorders. These issues are most often raised in reference to developmental apraxia of speech because children with this disorder rarely demonstrate obvious or "hard" signs of neurological dysfunction. Perhaps the most important issue to be addressed is: "What signs of motor impairment will I accept as characteristic of developmental apraxia of speech?" The answer to this question will depend on the beliefs of the questioner. If a unitary concept of developmental apraxia of speech is supported, clinicians may accept only poor performance on the more traditional tasks of isolated oral movements. This would be an unfortunate scenario because we know there are children with a severe apraxia of speech who demonstrate few or no signs of oral apraxia as evaluated by the more traditional tasks. Conversely, clinicians could subscribe to the perspective presented in Chapter 3 that motor performance, and hence motor impairment, is organized into functional subsystems along a continuum. From this perspective, the child with poor performance on movement sequences also may be considered apraxic, but with a different pattern of performance than the child with poor performance on both isolated and sequenced tasks. This approach bypasses the labeling issue by focusing more on the pattern of performance with the implication that underlying processes are reflected by performance on various tasks.

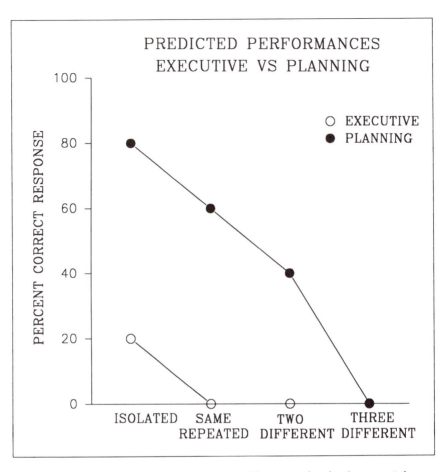

Figure 5-2. Predicted motor performance profiles across levels of sequential complexity in executive versus planning forms of apraxia.

Limb Motor Performance

Limb Apraxia: Basic Observations

Few studies of limb movement performance in children with apraxia of speech have been reported. However, many of the issues discussed in the section on oral motor performance are relevant to the discussion of limb motor performance. Many children with developmental motor speech disorders are considered to demonstrate signs of limb apraxia. Gubbay (1978) and Cermak (1985) separately noted that speech deficits frequently accompany limb apraxia in children. Aram and Horwitz (1983) observed that children with apraxia of speech often had difficulty learning sign language, presumably due to difficulties with learned manual skills. Dewey and colleagues (1988) reported that children with poor sequential motion speech performances (believed to

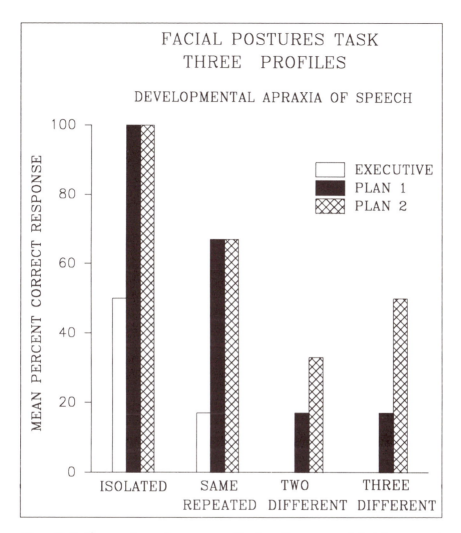

Figure 5–3. Three motor performance profiles from the nonspeech facial movement task representing executive versus planning forms of apraxia.

demonstrate an apraxia of speech) scored significantly lower on tests of limb praxis than normal-speaking controls or speech-disordered children who did not demonstrate impaired sequential motion speech abilities (nonpraxic speech deficit). Crary and Towne (1984) reported that children with apraxia of speech demonstrated similar performance deficits of tasks of oral and limb movement.

Parallels to Oral Motor Performance

Results of studies of limb movement deficits in children with apraxia of speech have paralleled those of oral movement deficits. Specifically, not all children demonstrate limb movement deficits, and there may be a decrease in performance as complexity of the attempted movement or movement sequence increases. Unfortunately, the few studies that have evaluated volitional limb motor performance have used different procedures. Often the procedures utilized seem unrelated to any theoretical orientation to the motor speech disorder. Aram and Horwitz (1983) assessed "manual gestures" using the Manual Expression subtest of the *Illinois Test of Psycholinguistic Ability* (Kirk, McCarthy, & Kirk, 1968). This procedure requires the child to pantomime the use of common objects such as binoculars, guitar, pencil sharpener, and so on. These movements reflect singular pantomimes as there is no systematic requirement for sequential movement patterns. Also, they are considered transitive movements because they relate to specific objects. Finally, they are "semantically potent" movements because a child must possess a degree of understanding of the characteristics of each object tested. Using this procedure, Aram and Horwitz found no significant performance deviations among children with apraxia of speech. They also evaluated performances on two construction praxis tasks: block design and object assembly. Similar to the results on the manual expression task, they found no significant performance deviations on these praxis tasks among children with apraxia of speech.

Dewey and her colleagues (1988) studied performance on both transitive and intransitive movements (movements not related to object use, such as waving goodbye) and included both single movements and two- and three-gesture movement sequences. For transitive movements, they evaluated performance both with and without the actual object. Finally, they evaluated performance on a motor sequencing task requiring children to learn a sequence of actions performed by moving a series of knobs. Their results were opposite of those of Aram and Horwitz (1983). Children with apraxia of speech differed from normal-speaking controls and nonapraxic speech impaired children on several parameters of limb apraxia. They did not differ in their ability to learn individual movements on the motor sequencing task, but they did complete significantly shorter sequences than the other groups. They performed poorer on both the individual and sequential movement limb tasks for both transitive and intransitive movements. However, when the actual object was provided for transitive movements, the performance of the speech apraxic group improved to the point where there was no difference between them and the other groups. None of these children had any difficulty recognizing gestures, implying that the observed movement deficits were the result of motor planning and/or execution. Dewey et al. suggested that examining motor sequencing abilities in different modalities was useful to differentiate performance profiles associated with various types of speech-language disorders including developmental motor speech disorders.

Perspectives from the Motolinguistic Model

The Aram and Dewey studies used different procedures and reached different conclusions regarding limb apraxia in children with developmental apraxia of speech. Should all children with a developmental apraxia of speech be expected to demonstrate an accompanying limb apraxia? The answer already provided is "no." Because both studies evaluated relatively small numbers of children, the discrepant results may represent the sampling process. The studies also used different procedures, and the discrepancies could reflect the adequacy of the procedures used to evaluate limb apraxia. Perhaps, as suggested by the motolinguistic model, limb apraxia should be evaluated by a series of motor tasks increasing systematically in sequential complexity. This strategy would not only facilitate the identification of volitional limb movement deficits, but also reveal the pattern of these deficits across varying levels of performance. The reports from Crary and Towne (1984) and Crary and Anderson (1990) were designed in reference to this model and did evaluate performance differences on limb movement tasks across levels of sequential complexity.

Both studies reported an increase in mean error rate as the sequential complexity of the limb movement task increased. The limb movement task used in both of these studies was a modification of the "fist-edge-palm" task described by Luria (1980). These three hand postures were performed in isolation, in a sequence of three repetitions of the same posture, in a sequence of two different postures, and in a sequence of three different postures. These postures or movements would be considered intransitive because they do not relate to specific objects and nonrepresentational because they convey no overt meaning. As seen in Figure 5–4, the expected performance decline with increasing sequential complexity of the stimuli was obtained.

Similar to the results of the oral movement task, these results may be interpreted to indicate sequencing difficulties. However, like the oral movement task results, analyses of error patterns do not support this position (Table 5–2). Again, the majority of the errors were designated as "groping" (trial-and-error searching movements with the fingers or hand). Very few errors of sequential order were identified. These data lend more support to the performance load explanation than to the sequential processing deficit position.

Similar to his evaluation of oral movement error profiles, Crary (1991) analyzed patterns of performance in reference to executive versus planning profiles of movement breakdown in the hand task. Recall the predicted pattern of performance associated with each type presented in Figure 5–2. Performance profiles from three children are presented in Figure 5–5. Like the oral movement task results, differing patterns of performance may be seen that match the predictions of the motolinguistic model associated with executive versus planning forms of apraxic impairment.

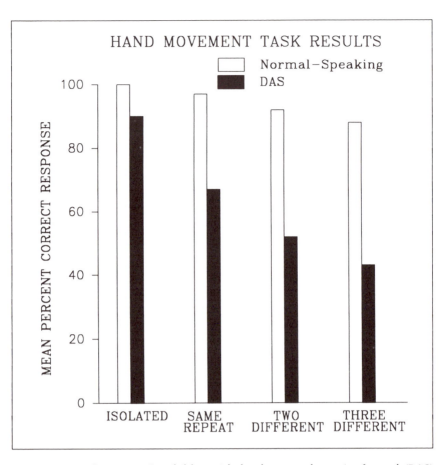

Figure 5–4. Performance of 10 children with developmental apraxia of speech (DAS) compared to 10 normal-speaking children of the same age on the task of volitional hand movements. (Data from Crary & Anderson, 1990)

Table 5–2. Hierarchy of error types for children with apraxia of speech and normal-speaking controls on a hand movement task. Ranking is from most to least frequent error type.

Ranking	Apraxic Group	Control Group
1	Groping	Incomplete posture
2	Slow release	Groping
3	Slow initiation	Slow release
4	Incomplete posture	Perseveration
5	Partial response	Added posture
6	Perseveration	Incorrect sequence
7	Use of hand	Slow transition
8	Slow transition	
9	Incorrect sequence	

Source: Data from Crary and Anderson (1990)

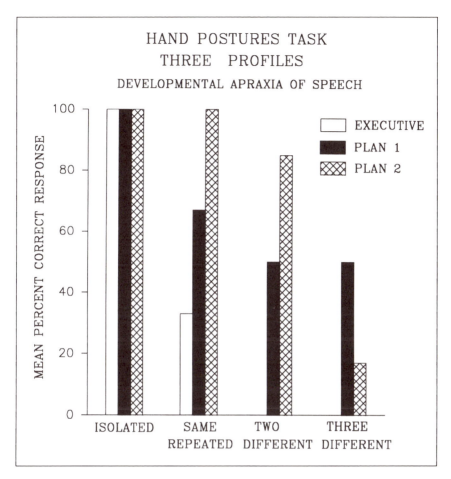

Figure 5–5. Three motor performance profiles from the hand movement task representing executive versus planning forms of apraxia.

Clinical Considerations

The results from the hand postures' task in the Crary series raise some interesting questions. There appears to be a high degree of similarity between performances on the oral task and the hand task. Both would implicate a performance deficit that is exaggerated with increased sequential complexity of attempted movements. One clinical implication of this finding is that frequently, but not always, when deficits in both areas are present, clinicians might expect a parallel pattern of performance in oral and limb movement tasks. This type of information could influence the choice of treatment strategies for the child with a developmental motor speech disorder. The performance of limb motor tasks by children with developmental motor speech disorders has not received as much attention as oral movement abilities; however, in individual cases this information may be as important or more important to successful case management.

Motor Speech Performance

Basic Observations

Speech is a complex motor act. Yet, meaningful speech production is also the result of complex linguistic processes. In this regard, when we discuss "motor speech performance" it is necessary to limit the scope of the discussion, often operationally and not without dissention. There is little argument that the various dysarthrias *are* motor speech disorders. In reference to developmental dysarthria, both Morley and her colleagues (1954) and Worster-Drought (1974) implicated anatomically focal weakness (i.e., lips, tongue, palate) as the direct cause of specific sound errors in speech production. Unfortunately, there has been little documentation of the characteristics of this developmental motor speech disorder. For example, does speech performance vary across different tasks? How severe are the basic motor deficits presumed to cause the overt speech production deficits? Does the speech pattern change over time? Are disturbances of movement and tone, other than weakness, responsible for the deviant speech dimensions?

Unanswered questions are even more prolific in the realm of developmental apraxia of speech. Because this speech disorder is envisioned by many as a "motor planning" disorder, no correspondence is expected between peripheral motor impairments and specific sound errors. If meaningful speech is used to evaluate motor speech performance, the picture is clouded by the addition of linguistic processing factors. Three investigative strategies have been used in attempts to evaluate the motor speech performance of children with developmental apraxia of speech. The least common of these approaches is the use of acoustic analysis to infer evidence of phonetic, presumably motoric, errors in speech. This strategy will be discussed further in the following chapter on speech performance. A second strategy, often used clinically, but with limited experimental validation, is the use of speech gymnastics tasks. These procedures typically require a child to repeat long, complicated polysyllabic words. The third and most common approach is the use of speech diadochokinetic tasks or the infamous "puh-tuh-kuh" procedure.

Speech Gymnastics

Morley (1965), Rosenbek and Wertz (1972), Yoss and Darley (1974a) and Aram and Glasson (1979) have reported that children with apraxia of speech have more difficulty, that is, make more errors, as word length increases. Many clinical procedures have taken these observations to heart. In their subtest for speech apraxia (not specific to children), Dworkin and Culatta (1980) request repeated repetitions of vowel sequences, the sequence "mommy-daddy-baby," and the repetition of polysyllabic words including "impossibility," "catastrophe," and "statistical analysis." In Blakeley's (1980) test for developmental apraxia of speech, children are asked to repeat three motorically complex words: "aluminum," "linoleum," and "statistics." They are judged on their ability to imitate the correct sound and syllable order. Additionally, this protocol asks children to imitate a variety of words that are provocative of transpositions, including "basket," "hamburger," "accident," "girl," and "nose." Productions are penalized for sound transpositions or syllable redundancies.

Each of these evaluation strategies appears to place great emphasis on the sequential aspects of speech production; however, the emphasis seems to be on sequencing rather than performance on systematically increased sequences. Furthermore, it is not clear whether such procedures have significant theoretical or clinical application to developmental motor speech disorders. They seem to offer little in the way of differential diagnosis, and they contribute little to the clinician's ability to profile motor performances across modalities. When a child is asked to produce a presumed motorically complex sequence of syllables, a variety of analyses may be completed. Verbal ordering or sequencing of the syllables, articulatory accuracy, prosodic features, and, last but not least, speed and "regularity" of the production may be noted. It would be beneficial to use a procedure that had some degree of comparable normative data and could be modified to test various components of the motor speech system. Finally, it would be a bonus if that procedure could be implemented simply. Possibly for these and other reasons, tests of speech diadochokinesis have been widely used in the evaluation of motor speech disorders in both children and adults.

Speech Diadochokinesis

Two basic methods are used to evaluate performance on speech diadochokinetic tasks: counting the number of syllables produced in a fixed time frame (count-by-time) or measuring the time it takes to produce a fixed number of syllables or syllable sequences (time-by-count). The second method, popularized by Fletcher (1972), asks the child to produce a specific number of syllables and syllable sequences while the clinician notes the production time on a stop watch. Possibly due to its simplicity, this procedure is widely used for evaluation of speech diadochokinetic performance.

Tests of speech diadochokinesis have become a central issue in the assessment of developmental motor speech disorders, especially developmental apraxia of speech. Yoss and Darley (1974a) reported that alternate motion rate tasks, such as repetition of the syllable "kuh," were performed more slowly by children demonstrating characteristics of apraxia of speech. Sequential motion rate tasks, such as repetition of the syllable sequence "puh-tuh-kuh," were performed even more slowly and with more difficulty, if they were completed at all. Aram and Glasson (1979) reported frequent difficulty with performance of alternate motion rate speech tasks in their apraxic group. Furthermore, none of the eight children described in their report was able to produce the "puh-tuh-kuh" sequence successfully. These findings led Aram to include difficulty or inability to complete these tasks as part of the diagnostic profile of the child with developmental apraxia of speech (Aram & Horwitz, 1983; Aram & Nation, 1982). Ludwig (1983) also used speech diadochokinetic performance as part of her subject descriptors in a study of phonological performance in developmental apraxia of speech. Ludwig contrasted performance among three groups of children: a group with developmental apraxia of speech, a group of normal-speaking children matched to the apraxic group based on receptive language ability, and a group of normal-speaking children matched to the apraxic group on expressive language ability. Because the apraxic group demonstrated an expressive-receptive language "split" with age-appropriate receptive language and deficient expressive language, the language-matched groups were of different ages. The group matched on expressive language performance was, on average, 17 months younger than the other two groups. This age-split among the groups afforded the opportunity to examine potential developmental aspects of diadochokinetic performance in children with apraxia of speech. The averaged data are presented in Table 5–3 for both the alternate motion tasks (AMR) (20 repetitions of each syllable) and the sequential motion task (SMR) (10 repetitions of the syllable sequence). The time-by-count method was used for analysis.

Table 5–3. Speech diadochokinesis results from 10 children with apraxia of speech, 10 normal-speaking children matched on expressive language ability and 10 normal-speaking children matched on receptive language ability. Group means and standard deviations ( ) are presented.

Group	Age (years;months)	P (sec)	T (sec)	K (sec)	PTK (sec)
Apraxic					
M	5;7	6.3	6.5	7.7	26.6
SD		(1.6)	(2.2)	(2.6)	(3.0)
Receptive language matched					
M	5;7	4.8	4.7	5.1	10.8
SD		(.81)	(1.1)	(.73)	(3.3)
Expressive language matched					
M	4;2	5.5	4.7	5.1	9.8
SD		(1.5)	(1.5)	(1.2)	(3.5)
Fletcher (1972) Norms					
M	6;0	4.8	4.9	5.5	10.3
SD		(1.0)	(1.0)	(1.0)	(2.8)

Note: The time-by-count method was used. Data are presented in number of seconds for 20 repetitions of the alternate motion tasks (P, T, and K) and 10 repetitions of the sequential motion task (PTK).

Source: Data from Ludwig (1983)

These data suggest that the children demonstrating developmental apraxia of speech were slower than either group of normal-speaking children in their performance of all diadochokinetic speech tasks. The greatest similarity among the three groups was seen on the alternate motion tasks ("P," "T," and "K"), and the greatest discrepancy was noted for the sequential motion task ("P-T-K"). Ludwig noted additional differences between the apraxic and normal-speaking groups on these tasks. Specifically, she reported that only 2 of the 10 apraxic speaking children could complete the required 10 repetitions of the SMR task. This performance deficit was in direct contrast to the normal-speaking groups. Among the children matched for receptive language ability (same age), none had any difficulty completing these tasks. Among those matched for expressive language ability (younger), only two children could *not* complete the SMR procedure. Thus, Ludwig's findings indicate that children demonstrating developmental apraxia of speech are quantitatively and qualitatively different from age-matched (receptive language) children and children nearly 1½ years young-er (expressive match) on tasks of speech diadochokinesis.

Perspectives from the Motolinguistic Model

Initial Performance Comparisons

The study by Crary and Anderson (1990) further examined performance of children with developmental apraxia of speech on tasks of speech diadochokinesis. These investigators used portions of Fletcher's (1972) procedure to compare speech diadochokinetic performance between children with developmental apraxia of speech and normal-speaking, age-matched controls. The speech tasks included 20 repetitions each of the isolated syllables "puh," "tuh," and "kuh"; 15 repetitions of the disyllables "puh-tuh" and "tuh-kuh"; and 10 repetitions of the trisyllable "puh-tuh-kuh." Three analyses were completed on the performances: number of subjects in each group who could complete the tasks, number of repetitions that were produced for each task regardless of successful completion, and the "speed" of production measured acoustically as intersyllabic duration in centiseconds. Table 5–4 presents the number of subjects in each group who successfully completed the respective tasks and the average number of repetitions per child in each group regardless of successful completion.

At this level of analysis there is little difference between disordered- and normal-speaking children for isolated bilabial and apical tasks. Velar productions ("kuh") reveal small differences that grow larger with the introduction of disyllabic tasks. However, the most notable difference between the groups was in the production of the trisyllabic sequence. None of the apraxic subjects was able to produce successfully this sequence. In fact, only 4 of the 10 subjects were able to produce correctly any trisyllabic responses. The mean number of productions for this group was 2.5 repetitions of the required 10 repetitions. An informal descriptive investigation of subjects' responses was

Table 5–4. Descriptive analysis of speech diadochokinetic performance by 10 children with apraxia of speech and 10 normal-speaking children of the same age.

| Task | Number of Children Completing Task | | Mean Number of Repetitions per Child | | |
	Apraxic	Control	Target	Apraxic	Control
P	10	10	20	20	20
T	10	10	20	20	20
K	9	10	20	18.1	20
PT	9	10	15	13.6	15
TK	7	9	15	10.3	14.4
PTK	0	9	10	2.5	9.1

Source: Data from Crary and Anderson (1990)

completed to determine whether the pattern of errors reflected sequencing deficits or deficits in producing longer sequences. Evidence supporting a sequencing deficit would have included production of all three syllables but in the wrong order. This was rarely, if ever, noted. The most prominent error type would be best described as perseveration. That is, the children with apraxia of speech would provide repetitions that persevervated on a given syllable such as "puh-puh-tuh" or "puh-tuh-tuh."

Speech timing analyses from these tasks also identified differences between the two groups of children. Specifically, the apraxic speakers were slower than the normal speakers on all of the speech diadochokinetic tasks. Furthermore, as the sequential complexity of the speech tasks increased the differences between the groups also increased (Figure 5–6).

Crary and Anderson (1990) summarized these findings in obvious terms. Few children with developmental apraxia of speech were able to complete all of the speech diadochokinetic tasks, specifically the sequential tasks. Children who could produce some of the sequential tasks produced fewer repetitions per attempt. As a group and individually the children with apraxia of speech demonstrated slower rates of production for all speech diadochokinetic tasks with their differences from normal-speaking children expanding as the sequential complexity of the task increased. Patterns of performance did not implicate a sequencing disorder per se. Rather, a deficit in the performance of sequentially complex units was implicated.

Patterns of Performance: Executive and Planning Profiles

Crary (1991) analyzed these data in reference to the motolinguistic model. Figure 5–7 displays the results of 10 control subjects in comparison to 2 children with apraxia of speech, 1 considered to present an executive deficit profile and 1 considered to present a planning deficit profile. The child with the executive profile produced slower diadochokinetic rates (i.e., greater num-

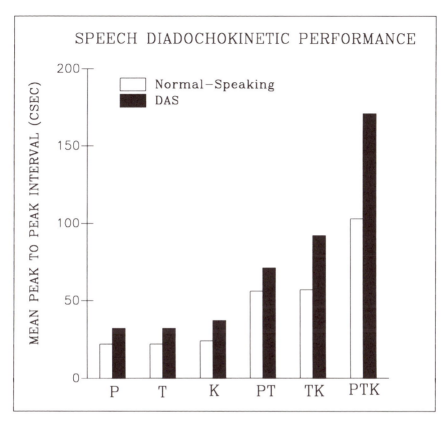

Figure 5-6. Performance of 10 children with developmental apraxia of speech (DAS) compared to 10 normal-speaking children of the same age on speech diadochinetic tasks. The data are presented as intersyllabic intervals in centiseconds. Higher values indicate slower diadochokinetic rates. (Data from Crary & Anderson, 1990)

ber of seconds to complete the task) than both the child with the planning deficit profile and the control group for the alternate motion tasks ("P," "T," and "K"). This child was unable to complete the sequential motion task ("P-T-K"). The child with the planning profile was slightly slower than the control group on the bilabial alternating task ("P"). There was a greater difference on the lingual alternating tasks ("T" and "K"), and a very pronounced difference on the sequential motion task ("P-T-K"). These findings match the profiles predicted by the motolinguistic model.

Clinical Reality

All experienced clinicians will realize the difficulties inherent in evaluating speech diadochokinetic abilities in children with speech articulation deficits. A common limitation is seen in the child who does not correctly produce one

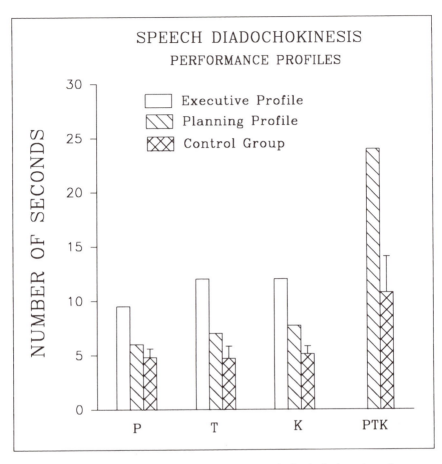

Figure 5–7. Three performance profiles from speech diadochokinetic tasks representing executive versus planning forms of apraxia compared to normal-speaking controls.

or more of the consonants used in the tasks. Also relevant to the motolinguistic model is the child who does not fit nicely into one end or the other of the continuum but demonstrates a mixed profile across various motor tasks. Both of these observations represent the reality of clinical practice—few clinical findings fit into neat clinical niches. Figure 5–8 demonstrates both of these possibilities as they relate to speech diadochokinesis performance.

These data are based on data from Crary and Anderson (1990). The measure of speech diadochokinetic performance in that study was intersyllabic duration in centiseconds. The longer the intersyllabic duration, the slower the diadochokinetic performance for the respective speech tasks. Each of the three children with apraxia of speech was "typed" (planning vs. executive) by his performance on the facial movement task. According to predictions from the motolinguistic model, their performances on the speech task should be

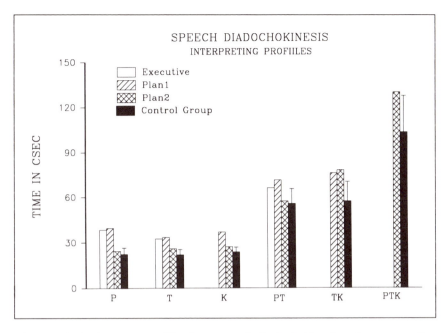

Figure 5–8. Performance profiles from speech diadochokinetic tasks representing executive versus planning forms of apraxia. Cases "executive" and "plan1" reflect clinical variations that may be encountered. The data are presented as intersyllabic intervals in centiseconds.

similar to their performances on the nonspeech task (i.e., they should have an executive or planning profile). This prediction, for the most part, is upheld, but there are deviations. Note that the executive case is unable to produce /k/, thus there are no data for "kuh" repetitions or for "tuh-kuh" or "puh-tuh-kuh." Yet, this child still is considered to demonstrate an executive profile because his productions of the remaining speech tasks were slower than the control group in all cases. The child identified as Plan2 seems to fall clearly within the planning range of the continuum. This child's alternate motion rate performances were similar to those of the control group while the sequential motion rate performances were slower. The child designated as Plan1 was considered to demonstrate a planning variant of apraxia based on performances on the facial movement task; however, on the speech diadochokinetic tasks, this child demonstrated more of an executive deficit profile. Performances on alternate motion rate tasks were slower than Plan2 and the control group, and there is a deterioration of performance on sequential motion tasks with inability to perform the trisyllabic sequence. Because Plan1 has some characteristics of both executive and planning deficits, the most appropriate designation might be "mixed." Other factors might be helpful in determining whether one deficit profile is more prominent than the other. In this instance, a review of performances on the face and hand tasks revealed that Plan1 demonstrated a profile similar to Plan2 but made more errors on each task. Based on performance profiles from the respective motor tasks (including speech), Plan1 was considered to demonstrate a severe planning apraxia.

Beyond Diadochokinesis: Bite Block Basics

Speech diadochokinesis is a common and useful clinical approach to evaluation of motor speech abilities. Still, at times, it may be important or even necessary to "stress" the entire motor speech mechanism to provide a more thorough evaluation. Clinicians can stress the mechanism by asking the child to increase rate or loudness or by pushing the child's ability to maximum performance levels (Kent, Kent, & Rosenbek, 1987). Another method of taxing the system is to introduce a disruptor that alters the usual and expected manner of speech production. One such technique that has been used to study both normal and abnormal speech is to stabilize the mandible during speech via placement of a bite block between the maxillary and mandibular teeth.

According to Kelso and Tuller (1983), "a well-established feature of speech production is that talkers, faced with either anticipated or unanticipated perturbations, can spontaneously adjust the movement patterns of articulators such that the acoustic output remains relatively undistorted" (p. 217). Normal-speaking adults (Fowler & Turvey, 1980; Gay, Lindblom, & Lubker, 1981; Kelso & Tuller, 1983) and children with normal articulation (Baum & Katz, 1988) and disordered articulation (DeJarnette, 1988) compensate immediately on vowels produced with a bite block stabilizing the jaw. Adult patients with Broca's aphasia, however, do not seem to compensate well for this perturbation. Sussman, Marquardt, Hutchinson, and MacNeilage (1986) reported that aphasic patients not only demonstrated a consistent inability to compensate for the presence of a bite block during vowel production, but that this limitation in compensatory ability was strongly related to the severity of oral apraxia. They speculated that areas of the left hemisphere felt to be important in motor speech control may contribute to the ability to compensate for bite block interference during speech production. Crary, Hardy, and Williams (1985) described an adult patient with an apraxia of speech who demonstrated limitations in his ability to compensate for bite block perturbation in the absence of any measurable sensorimotor limitations in the oral mechanism. This patient had a small focal lesion within the left hemisphere in the superior aspect of Broca's area and the inferior precentral gyrus. Similar to Sussman et al. (1986) these investigators implied that the patient's difficulty in compensating for bite block interference (they used a speech diadochokinetic task) was related to observed apraxia of speech secondary to the left inferior frontal lobe lesion.

Crary, Turner, and Williams (1990) described performances of three adults with motor speech disorders on speech diadochokinetic tasks with and without bite block interference. They also studied lingual-mandibular relationships on a nonspeech fine motor task. Each of these patients had suffered left hemisphere damage and was considered to demonstrate only a mild aphasia in the presence of speech production deficits. Two of the patients were felt to demonstrate an executive form of apraxia. The third was felt to demonstrate a planning variant based on face and hand movement tasks. One interesting observation from their data is that little difference from a group of normal controls was observed on any of the alternate motion rate tasks when no bite block was used. Speech diadochokinetic performances in the three patients deteriorated with the introduction of a bite block. This was not seen in a control group. The interference effects were not equivalent across tasks and patients. The executive patients demonstrated reduced performances for both alternate and sequential motion rates. The patient designated as planning demonstrated an interference effect only for the sequential motion rate task. Using a strain-gauge system designed to simultaneously measure lingual protrusive and mandibular bite forces, these investigators demonstrated that their three subjects were able to perform nonspeech lingual fine motor tasks within normal limits. However, these normal lingual motor performances were accompanied by abnormally high levels of mandibular activity. Their findings were interpreted to show that an abnormal level of mandibular support was required to accomplish a normal lingual fine motor performance. This pattern may explain why speech diadochokinetic rates differed from a control group only when a bite block, removing potential mandibular support, was used to stabilize the mandible.

Virtually nothing is known about motor biomechanics in children with disordered speech. Dworkin (1978) has suggested the use of a bite block in therapy to facilitate improved lingual-alveolar valving during speech production. His premise is that some children with speech disorders have excessive mandibular activity during speech. DeJarnette (1988) reported that children with moderate speech articulation disorders were able to compensate for bite block interference during vowel production. However, the simple vowel production task used in that study may have been insufficient to elicit changes in the speech pattern. Towne and Melgren (1987) reported that a combined group of children with and without speech disorders demonstrated slower speech diadochokinetic rates when a bite block was used to stabilize the jaw. Furthermore, they suggested that the interference effect did not seem to be related to the presence or absence of a phonological disorder. Unfortunately, a major limitation in their study was the lack of direct comparison between speech-normal and speech-disordered subjects. Also, there was no indication of the type of speech problems included in their group other than that the children were receiving speech therapy.

Clinical Implications

If bite block interference, or more specifically a speech disordered child's ability to compensate for bite block interference, is to become a useful clinical tool in the evaluation of developmental motor speech disorders, additional studies are needed. The information currently available to clinicians comes primarily from limited reports based on adults with normal or disordered speech. However, clinicians may apply these principles to the evaluation of developmental motor speech disorders if they are willing to allow for the significant gaps in knowledge.

At this juncture we are left with a few incomplete principles that might be applicable to developmental motor speech disorders. The more important of these principles include: (1) Deviations in speech diadochokinetic performance may be minimal until a bite block is used to reduce mandibular support during the speech tasks; and (2) The pattern of interference seen on speech diadochokinetic tasks resulting from jaw stabilization via a bite block may indicate underlying deficits in motor speech control. These speculations are based on few observations. At the very least, however, this technique might be used clinically to evaluate the presence of "lingual-mandibular dependency" and its potential contribution to the overt speech disorder (Dworkin, 1978; Towne & Melgren, 1987).

Relationships Among Motor Indices

Predictions from the Motolinguistic Model

The motolinguistic model implies potential relationships among the various motor indices: face movement, limb (hand) movement, and speech (diadochokinesis). More specifically, the model predicts that, when deficits in face, limb, and speech motor performances are present, they will reveal parallel patterns of performance. For example, because the dysarthria associated with congenital suprabulbar paresis is the result of focal corticobulbar deficits, we would not expect to find limb motor deficits in pure instances of this disorder. If limb motor deficits were present, we might expect that, similar to observed facial motor deficits, they would reflect upper motor neuron weakness (spastic paresis). Among children with apraxia of speech, the frequent coexistence of deficits in face, hand, and speech motor indices would seem to support the position that they are, in fact, the result of a deficit in a common underlying mechanism. This view of the apraxias posits that distinctions among output modalities may be artificial. Coexistence of deficits in various output modalities and similarity of error types across output modalities are often used to argue for this position (Roy & Square, 1985). Kimura (1976) felt that a common neural system governed speech, oral and limb movements. Conversely, Raade, Rothi, and Heilman (1991) in a study of oral and limb apraxia argued against the unitary position. They concluded that oral and limb apraxias "were not significantly associated, were differentially influenced by the nature of the movement . . ., exhibited different proportions of error types, and demonstrated different neuroanatomy" (p. 141). Their position is that these modality variants of apraxia are functionally independent.

Chapter 3 presented information suggesting a strong functional and neuroanatomic relationship between speech and oral motor control relative to the apraxias. This implied relationship seems quite logical, and evidence that supports a special relation between these two motor functions is mounting. Limb motor functions may be the odd man out. This distinction is not trivial. There are important theoretical and clinical implications and applications to understanding potential relationships among these three motor indices. For example, Dewey et al. (1988) felt that children with disordered speech who demonstrated a more generalized motor impairment (including deficits on limb motor tasks) may represent a verbal apraxia (authors' term). However, children who did not demonstrate limb deficits but did demonstrate oral motor deficits were felt to represent a phonological or language-based problem. On the other extreme of this scenario, Aram and Horwitz (1983) reported that, as a group, children demonstrating developmental verbal apraxia did not present manual-gestural or constructional apraxias.

Checking the Predictions: Measuring Relationships

The motolinguistic model implies that there may be some relationships among speech, face, and hand movement deficits. To study these potential interrelations, Crary and Anderson (1990) computed correlations among the three motor indices based on data from their 20 subjects (disordered and control combined). These data are presented in Table 5–5.

To identify descriptive trends in relationships among face, hand and motor speech performances, Crary and Anderson calculated the average of all of the correlations between two respective variables. The highest average correlation was obtained from the comparison of results from the face and hand tasks (.51). The next highest average correlation was obtained between the face and speech diadochokinetic tasks (−.41). The lowest average correlation was obtained between the speech diadochokinetic and hand task results (−.32). None of these average correlations are strikingly high. At best, the relationships would be described as moderate to weak. Somewhat stronger correlations were obtained when comparing the three motor indices to speech articulation ability as measured by the *Templin-Darley Screening Test of Articulation* (Templin & Darley, 1960). From these comparisons, the face task results produced the highest average correlation (.77), followed by the speech diadochokinesis results (−.63), and, in last place, the hand task results (.43). Collectively, these findings suggest that results of the hand movement task correlated poorly with both speech performance indexes (articulation test or speech diadochokinesis). In each case, the face task results demonstrated a stronger relationship. Yet, there was a moderate relationship between the face and the hand task results. These findings are important in depicting a

Table 5-5. Summary of correlations among articulation test scores, speech diadochokinetic (intersyllabic interval in csec), nonspeech facial (percent correct response), and hand movement (percent correct response) data from the combined 20 subjects. Values rounded.

	TD	P	T	K	PT	TK	PTK	H1	H2	H3	H4
TD		−.65	−.61	−.59	−.55	−.62	−.73				
F1	.59	−.27	−.41	−.29	−.24	−.29	−.37	.06	.71	.62	.50
F2	.77	−.40	−.62	−.51	−.52	−.61	−.47	.18	.54	.78	.68
F3	.89	−.46	−.56	−.45	−.57	−.46	−.69	.04	.42	.74	.63
F4	.84	−.42	−.73	−.62	−.60	−.68	−.60	.30	.53	.69	.75
H1	.00	−.01	−.46	−.36	−.27	−.12	−.18				
H2	.44	−.24	−.33	−.24	−.34	−.24	−.67				
H3	.65	−.29	−.38	−.27	−.20	−.10	−.50				
H4	.63	−.36	−.66	−.60	−.38	−.38	−.14				

Note: TD = Templin-Darley Screening Test of Articulation. P, T, K, PT, TK, and PTK represent the respective speech diadochokinetic tasks. F1-F4 and H1-H4 represent the four sequential complexity levels of the face (F) and hand (H) tasks, respectively.

Source: Data from Crary and Anderson (1990)

motor performance profile for children with apraxia of speech. Not all children will demonstrate deficits in all three motor indexes; however, when deficits in two or more modalities are present, the motolinguistic model and the available data suggest that performances across modalities will be related.

Summary

Children with developmental motor speech disorders frequently present a variety of motor limitations beyond the speech production deficit. The child with dysarthria, by definition, would be expected to demonstrate abnormal oral reflexes, vegetative functions, and spastic weakness in the oral musculature. The deviations in the child with an apraxia of speech are not anticipated to be so obvious. Among apraxic children, limitations in volitional motor performance may include nonspeech oral and/or limb movements. In many cases parallel patterns of performance would be expected across modalities. However, exceptions should be anticipated. Motor speech limitations, commonly evaluated via speech diadochokinetic tasks, are expected to reveal profiles similar to limitations in other, nonspeech motor performances. There may be instances when it will be necessary to stress the motor speech mechanism by using a bite block or other disruptor to reduce compensatory mechanisms before the pattern of motor limitations will become obvious. Finally, and most importantly, the majority of information regarding motor functions, including motor speech functions, in children with developmental motor speech disorders is based on very small numbers of children or on predictions based on performances of adults with motor speech disorders. Clinicians are encouraged to incorporate these strategies into their clinical tool chest only with the caveat that knowledge is limited.

Think About This

The terms dysarthria and apraxia denote motor performance deviations. Yet, sparse knowledge exists describing motor performance characteristics of children with developmental motor speech disorders. Few truisms exist. A variety of observations do, however, provide small windows of insight that may be clinically helpful. These include but are not limited to:

1. Children with dysarthria secondary to congenital suprabulbar paresis should demonstrate signs of upper motor neuron involvement, and their speech errors are expected to be anatomically related to the observed weakness.
2. Different forms of apraxia of speech are expected to demonstrate different profiles of motor performance deficits.
3. Motor performance profiles in children with an apraxia of speech (and possibly dysarthria) are expected to be similar across modalities (oral, speech, limb) when deficits exist in more than one modality.
4. It may be necessary to stress the speech system (and possibly nonspeech and limb systems) to identify motor performance deficits.
5. **The type of procedure used to evaluate motor characteristics will influence the identification of motor performance profiles.**

These observations suggest potentially important clinical directions in the evaluation of children with developmental motor speech disorders. Like many observations focal to developmental motor speech disorders, they should be questioned and modified as new information is acquired. Optimism indicates that the situation is not clearly understood. Clinical reality dictates that expected patterns will not be followed closely. With this in mind, the predictions of the motolinguistic model and the preliminary data supporting these predictions should be viewed as general clinical guidelines rather than a specific menu.

CHAPTER

Six

Speech Performance

Traditionally, the clinical hallmark of developmental motor speech disorders has been a severe and persistent deficit in speech articulation abilities. The implication is that something has gone awry with various aspects of motor speech control that prohibits the development of speech production along expected routes and timelines. An important consideration in discussing speech performance is the manner in which the speech disorder is described. Different sources of description may well influence the characteristics attributed to the disorder. Theories and techniques applied to the description of disordered speech have changed vastly since the writings of Morley and Worster-Drought. These changes have influenced our perceptions of developmental motor speech disorders, if for no other reason than differences in the way characteristics of speech are portrayed. Crary and Fokes (1980) addressed the issue of different speech analysis techniques pertaining to concepts surrounding apraxia of speech in adults and concluded that perceptions of the disorder were dramatically influenced by the results obtained from different analysis techniques.

Many variables must be considered when evaluating speech characteristics of developmental motor speech disorders. This chapter will address some of these variables. Of particular interest will be the nature of speech analysis procedures used to reach conclusions regarding the various developmental motor speech disorders.

Changes in Latitudes—Changes in Attitudes

Sound Count Analyses

Two basic approaches to the analysis of speech have been used in recent history. The earlier and more traditional approach has been to make a list of individual sound errors produced by the child. This approach might be referred to as the "sound count approach." Errors were commonly classified as substitutions, omissions, distortions, or additions. Examples of this approach applied to developmental motor speech disorders may be seen in the writings of Morley and Worster-Drought. A common perception of the speech of children with developmental dysarthria was that errant speech sounds related directly to the paresis in the mechanism. Therefore, if the lips were weak, labial sounds would be erred; if the tongue was weak, lingual sounds would be erred; and so on. Although this approach has certain utility, it would seem limited in the presence of multiple speech errors that involved more than one point of articulation. It also would seem limited in explaining why children produced sounds correctly in some words but not in others. In short, this strict sound-by-peripheral-anatomy approach simply does not have much descriptive or explanatory power. Despite its limitations, variants of this approach were applied to the study of developmental motor speech disorders at least into the late 1970s. For example, Rosenbek and Wertz (1972) stated that phonemic errors were prominent in the speech of children with apraxia of speech, including omissions, substitutions, distortions, additions, repetitions, and prolongations. Aram and Glasson (1979) reported that younger children with apraxia of speech demonstrated a high vowel-to-consonant ratio and that omissions and substitutions were the dominant error patterns. These types of analyses focused attention on the sound level of speech production. This focus not only directed impressions of developmental apraxia of speech, but also influenced assessment and therapy strategies.

Phonological Analyses: The Organization of Sound Systems

During the 1970s a change in approach became evident. This change may be characterized as a growing influence from linguistic science that shifted emphasis away from a sound count and motor deficit approach to evaluating the organization of speech production systems. In simple terms, during this period the term phonological disorder began to have a significant influence on our perceptions of the nature of speech disorders in children. Two major approaches emerged with introduction of the more linguistic-based approaches to the assessment of speech articulation disorders: distinctive feature analysis and phonological process analysis. These techniques use different terminology and procedures, but both are intended to evaluate patterns in the apparent chaos of disordered speech systems. Yoss and Darley (1974a) were among the first to employ these techniques in the study of developmental apraxia of speech. They reported that the number of distinctive feature errors was a key consideration in differentiating children with apraxia of speech from children with other speech impairments. Crary (Crary, 1984b; Crary, Landess, & Towne, 1984) utilized phonological process analysis to describe error patterns in children with developmental apraxia of speech. The results of phonological analyses suggested that there was a systematic organization within the disordered phonological systems of apraxic children.

Factors Thought to Influence Speech Performance

Beyond consideration of the analysis system used to describe speech errors, clinicians must decide in which "environments" to evaluate speech performance. Environment might refer to any number of factors thought to influence speech performance. For example, some children may perform better in imitative tasks compared to conversational tasks; others may demonstrate deterioration in performance as the length of response increases. These two factors, imitation and length of response, are frequently cited as influential in the speech performance of the child with apraxia of speech (Morley, 1965; Rosenbek & Wertz, 1972, Yoss & Darley, 1974a). These factors also may influence speech performance in the dysarthric speaker (Morley, Court, & Miller, 1954; Yorkston, Beukelman, & Bell, 1988). Finally, these factors may interact in their influence on speech performance. For example, both Rosenbek and Wertz (1972) and Aram and Glasson (1979) reported that children with an apraxia of speech may be able to imitate certain speech sounds in isolation but not in sound sequences or "connected" speech. These observations suggest that different performance patterns may be obtained when different tasks are used to evaluate speech performance. Are differences in speech performance profiles obtained by different techniques? Is there a best way to evaluate speech performance? Are different conclusions reached by using different evaluation techniques? These and perhaps other issues should be considered when evaluating speech performance.

What Should Be Evaluated/Analyzed?

How microscopic should we be in the evaluation of speech errors? Aram and Nation (1982) pointed out that, with two exceptions (Aram & Glasson, 1979; Yoss & Darley, 1974a), there have been no attempts to differentiate between phonologic and phonetic characteristics of developmental apraxia of speech. Yet, only three studies have evaluated acoustic characteristics of speech produced by children with apraxia of speech (Crary & Towne, 1984; Glasson, 1981, 1984). Is the information gained from this level of analysis useful in understanding, evaluating, and/or differentiating developmental motor speech disorders?

Speech production is more than a simple string of sounds. Speech has an expected rhythm or melody that may be just as deviant as the errors in the segments themselves. Prosodic aspects of speech include not only rhythm and intonation patterns, but speech rate and syllabic stress patterns. Many investigators have commented on the prosodic irregularities noted in the speech of apraxic children. Unfortunately, to date, no data have been published describing prosodic characteristics of children with developmental motor speech disorders (apraxia or dysarthria).

Acoustic and/or prosodic analyses of speech production may provide a more complete, detailed description of speech performance in children with a developmental motor speech disorder. Comparisons along these dimensions may help to identify developmental motor speech disorders by delineating distinctions from other types of speech deficit. Such analyses also may assist in differentiating subtypes of developmental motor speech disorders.

Obviously, many gaps exist in our knowledge of speech performance in children with developmental motor speech disorders. A variety of descriptions are available that have been derived from multiple and differing procedures. The heterogeneity in techniques used to describe developmental motor speech disorders may well have contributed to the distribution of perceptions regarding these disorders. In this introduction, questions have been raised regarding analysis procedures and even the focus of analysis. The remainder of this chapter presents information on speech performance relevant to these questions. Phonologic, acoustic, and prosodic parameters of speech performance are described with consideration for the potential influences of imitation and performance load.

Speech Articulation/Phonological Performance

Anatomically Specific Errors in Dysarthria

Among cases of congenital suprabulbar paresis there are relatively pure developmental dysarthrias (i.e., no concomitant apraxias or language deficits). Such children may well develop an elaborate phonological system but demonstrate "anatomically specific" errors in speech production secondary to spastic paresis. Perhaps the most common example of this type of error is the child with excessive nasality in the presence of a structurally normal velopharynx. The straightforward nature of this speech deficit would be expected only in the incomplete form of congenital suprabulbar paresis, specifically, when the velopharyngeal musculature was affected in isolation. Children presenting the complete form of this disorder would be expected to demonstrate a more widespread articulation/phonological disorder just as they demonstrate a more widespread paresis in the speech musculature.

The Multitude of Errors in Apraxia of Speech

Speech performance characteristics of children with apraxia of speech have been studied in more detail than those of children with an isolated developmental dysarthria. From studies such as Morley (1965), Rosenbek and Wertz

(1972), Yoss and Darley (1974a), and Aram and Glasson (1979) several common findings may be extracted despite different procedures and purposes. Eight of these "common findings" are presented in Table 6-1. This list is not exhaustive; however, it does include many overlapping observations made in reference to speech performance in children with apraxia of speech. There appears to be a general consensus that these children (as well as dysarthric children) demonstrate a severe phonological disorder that is characterized by a restricted sound inventory. This restriction seems to be the result of a high percentage of omission errors. Yet, even among the sounds that are produced by these children, there is evidence of substitutions, sequencing errors (metathesis usually in the form of transposed sound sequences within words), and intrusions (additions). A consistent observation from all of these reports is the performance load factor. Simply stated, the performance load factor refers to the observation that more errors occur as production demands are increased. Increased performance load could result from attempting to produce sounds that require more complex articulatory adjustments, from increasing word length or length of utterance, and/or from differences between repetition and conversation tasks. Finally, abnormal prosodic features in speech production are frequently mentioned.

Although many of these observations depict a severe phonological disorder, only in the early 1980s did Crary and a variety of colleagues begin studying phonological organization in children with apraxia of speech. The initial questions were simple: (1) Is there a pattern of phonological errors in the speech of children with apraxia of speech? If so, how is it organized?; (2) What potential relationships exist between the phonological disorder and other language limitations? and (3) How is phonological performance influenced by performance load factors? Following is a review of the data used in attempts to answer each of the questions.

Table 6–1. Speech performance characteristics commonly reported in cases of developmental apraxia of speech.

Multiple speech sound errors representing omissions (most prominent), substitutions, additions, and distortions of consonants and vowels.

Difficulties with sound sequencing, including transposing sound sequences and inability to use sounds in sequences that are acceptable in isolation.

Errors increase as word length increases.

Single words are more intelligible than conversation.

Errors vary with the complexity of articulatory adjustment.

Errors are consistent.

Probable differences between repetition and conversation.

Prosodic aspects of speech are abnormal.

Phonological Processes: Patterns of Organization

A series of descriptive studies was completed for the purpose of identifying phonological processes prominent in the speech of children demonstrating an apraxia of speech (Crary, 1984b). Thirteen processes (Table 6-2) were selected for analyses based on literature available at that time (Hodson, 1980; Ingram, 1976; Shriberg & Kwiatkowski, 1980) with consideration for the "descriptive power" of the set of processes used. Crary (1982) evaluated these 13 phonological processes for their ability to account for the total number of errors in children's speech. Results indicated that this set accounted for an

Table 6-2. Thirteen phonological processes used in phonological descriptions of children with developmental apraxia of speech by Crary (1984b; Crary, Landess, & Towne, 1984).

Process	Definition/Description	Example
Deletion of Final Consonants (DFC)	Syllable final consonant deleted or replaced by a glottal stop	tap → ta tap → taʔ
Deletion of Initial Consonant (DIC)	Initial consonant omitted	kʌt → ʌt
Glottal Replacement (GR)	Oral consonant replaced by /ʔ/ or /h/. Deletion of intervocalic consonants	bebɪ → beʔɪ sʌn → hʌn pʌpɪ → pʌiː
Weak Syllable Deletion (WSD)	Unstressed syllable omitted from polysyllabic word	tɛləfon → tɛfon
Cluster Reduction (CR)	Consonant cluster simplified by omission or substitution	stap → tap ple → pe
Prevocalic Voicing (PVV)	Voiceless obstruent becomes voiced in the prevocalic position	to → do si → zi
Stopping (ST)	Fricatives or affricates replaced by stops	sʌn → tʌn tʃɛr → tɛr
Fronting (FR)	Velar or palatal sounds produced at a more frontal point of articulation	kʌp → tʌp go → do
Backing (BK)	Alveolar sound produced as a velar sound	toz → koz du → gu
Gliding (GL)	Liquids replaced by glides	rʌn → wʌn laɪt → jaɪt
Vocalization (VOC)	Syllablic /r/ or /l/ replaced by a full vowel	hæmr̩ → hæmu tebl̩ → tebo
Labialization (LAB)	Replacement of a lingual consonant by a labial consonant	ti → pi
Vowel Neutralization (VN)	Nonneutral vowel replaced by ʌ or ə	Any vowel → ʌ, ə

average of 84% of all errors with a range from 59% to 97%. Furthermore, the accountability or descriptive power of this set of phonological processes was significantly correlated with the severity of the phonological problem. Thus, as the severity of the problem increased, the accountability of the set of processes also increased.

To provide an objective index to the phonological process analysis, a ratio of the number of occurrences of each process to number of potential occurrences was used. This ratio, or percent of error, was termed the "relative strength" of the phonological process (number of occurrences divided by the number of potential occurrences = relative strength of process). Children were selected for these studies based on criteria consistent with published descriptions of apraxia of speech. Ages of the children varied from study to study, but the vast majority of the children in these collective studies were between the ages of 4 and 7 years.

Initially, three descriptive studies were completed. The first included 10 children, the second 25 children and the third reevaluated children in the second study, with individuals over 13 years of age deleted from the data base. Each of these studies produced strikingly similar results. The results of the third study are presented in Figures 6–1 and 6–2. The mean age of the children in the apraxic group in that study was 5;8 with a range from 3;11 to 13;0. Only 4 of the 20 children in this group were older than 7;6. To provide a comparison, equivalent data from 20 normally developing preschool children are presented. The mean age of these children was 3;11 with a range from 2;11 to 4;8. Figure 6–1 presents the number of children in each group demonstrating each of the respective phonological processes. Figure 6–2 presents the relative strength of the respective processes identified in each group.

The information in Figure 6–1 suggests that the same types of errors were made by both groups with a higher prevalence among the apraxic speakers. This is a misleading conclusion. Children with apraxia of speech, as a group, averaged 10.9 different error types (phonological processes). In fact, only 3 of the 20 apraxic children demonstrated fewer than 10 different error types and 6 children demonstrated 12 or 13 out of the 13 possible error types. A dramatically different result was obtained in the speech-language normal group. These children averaged 3.9 different error types and only four children demonstrated more than five different phonological processes. Figure 6–2 demonstrates that the average strength of the identified phonological processes was much less among the speech-language normal children. In these respects, two important findings emerge from these data: (1) Children with an apraxia of speech produced a greater variety of errors than children with normal speech-language performance; and (2) The apraxic group demonstrated more severe errors (a higher relative strength value) in all error categories. These results suggest that children with apraxia of speech differ in both type and severity of phonological errors from younger children with normal speech-language abilities. The results from the apraxic group also support prior reports in that

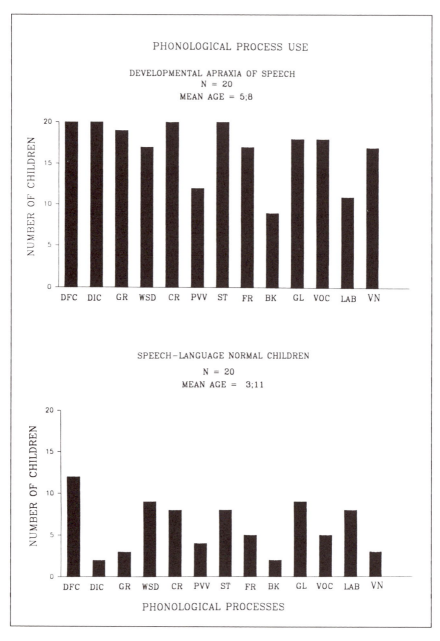

Figure 6–1. Comparison of the prevalence of phonological process use in 20 children with developmental apraxia of speech (top) versus 20 children with normal speech-language abilities (bottom).

the dominant errors were those of omission. Phonological processes resulting in syllabic structure simplification were among the most prevalent and in-

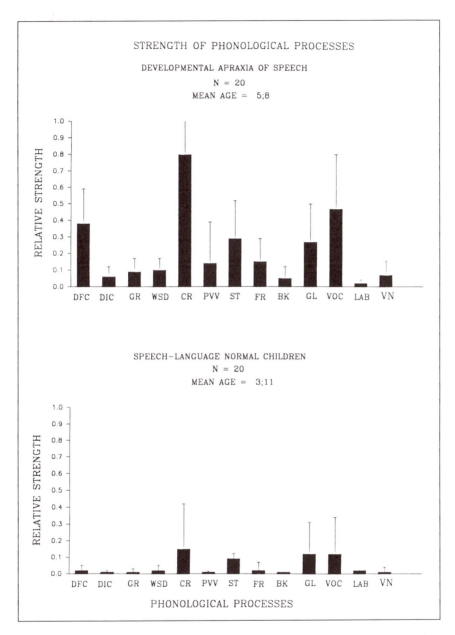

Figure 6–2. Comparison of the average error frequency (relative strength) of phonological processes in 20 children with developmental apraxia of speech (top) versus 20 children with normal speech-language abilities (bottom).

cluded the strongest errors. Manner of articulation errors involving fricative, affricative, and liquid sound classes also were prominent in this group. Errors of place of articulation were among the least frequent and weakest.

Sound Class Analysis: Bridging the Gap

From the initial phonological process analyses, it is obvious that no error oc-curred 100% of the time. This observation implies some selectivity among sound classes influenced by the respective processes. Because errors of omis-sion have been emphasized in developmental apraxia of speech, these pro-cesses were evaluated further with respect to manner and place features of sounds influenced by these processes. This analysis involved responses from 15 children with apraxia of speech to a phrase imitation task. The phrase imi-tation task was chosen to ensure that all of the subjects had attempted the same phonological targets.

Manner of Articulation

Table 6–3 presents the results of analysis of manner of articulation for three omission processes. Nasals and stops were, on average, the least omitted sound classes, whereas fricatives were omitted most frequently. The relative-ly high values for sonorant sounds for initial and final consonant deletion re-flect difficulty with /r/ and /l/ production.

Place of Articulation

Table 6–4 presents the results of analysis regarding place of articulation for the same three omission processes. Three places of articulation were analyzed: labial, tongue-front (apical), and tongue-back (palatal and velar). These re-sults clearly indicate that lingual sounds were omitted more often than labial sounds. A slight tendency was noted for apical sound to be omitted more than back sounds, especially in the syllable-initial position.

Cluster Errors

Cluster reduction was perhaps the single most dominant phonological pro-cess observed in the descriptive studies. All of the children with an apraxia of speech who were evaluated demonstrated difficulty with production of clus-ters at a very high error rate (average of 80%). Given the dominance of omis-sion errors, it was anticipated that clusters would be reduced primarily by

Table 6–3. Mean proportion of error (relative strength) for manner of articulation analysis of three phonological processes of omission.

	Manner of Articulation				
Process	Nasal	Stop	Fricative	Affricate	Sonorant
Delete Final Consonant	0.13	0.19	0.39	0.27	0.32
Delete Initial Consonant	0.02	0.03	0.04	0.02	0.06
Glottal Replacement	0.06	0.05	0.15	0.08	0.05
Mean	0.07	0.09	0.19	0.12	0.14

Source: Adapted from Crary (1984b).

Table 6-4. Mean proportion of error (relative strength) of three places of articulation for three phonological processes of omission.

| | Place of Articulation | | |
Process	Labial	Apical	Back
Delete Final Consonant	0.17	0.34	0.31
Delete Initial Consonant	0.08	0.16	0.04
Glottal Replacement	0.03	0.11	0.11
Mean	0.07	0.20	0.15

Source: Adapted from Crary (1984b).

omission of one or both of the sounds involved. Cluster errors were analyzed in reference to syllable shape and sound change. Only two-segment prevocalic clusters were analyzed. Table 6-5 presents the results of this analysis.

Four types of cluster errors were identified, accounting for 97% of all cluster errors. Type I errors are those in which one segment of the cluster is omitted but the other, original member remains. This changes the syllable shape of the word from CCVC to CVC (e.g., /stap → tap/). These were the most frequent errors, occurring 41% of the time. Type II errors are those in which one member of the cluster is substituted, but two segments are produced (e.g., /tren → twen/). These changes accounted for 23% of cluster errors. Type III errors involve production of a single consonant that was not part of the original cluster (e.g., /trʌk → dʌk/). These errors accounted for 29% of cluster errors. The least frequent cluster error, Type IV, accounted for only 4% of the errors. These productions resulted in a cluster containing two segments that were not in the original target (e.g., /krim → twim/). The remaining 3% of cluster errors identified were isolated instances in which the entire cluster was omitted or replaced by a laryngeal [h]. Obviously, the dominant type of cluster

Table 6-5. Analysis of cluster reduction errors.

Type of Error	Form	Percent of Occurrence
I	CVC	41
II	CC_sVC	23
III	C_nVC	29
IV	C_nC_nVC	4
Other	1. Omit	
	2. CC → [h]	3

Note: C = consonant, V = vowel, s = substitution, n = a new consonant that was not in the target word

Source: Adapted from Crary (1984b).

error involved omission of one segment of the target cluster. This error pattern accounted for 70% of all cluster errors (Type I and Type III combined).

Vowel Errors

Vowel errors also have been mentioned among the speech characteristics attributed to children with apraxia of speech. However, there seems to be wide variation among impressions regarding vowel errors in this group of children. Morley (1965) reported that vowels and diphthongs often were produced normally, but might be affected in severe cases, especially diphthongs. Rosenbek and Wertz (1972) felt that vowel errors were more prevalent among younger children with an apraxia of speech and the presence of vowel errors might be of diagnostic significance. Yoss and Darley (1974a) reported that they did not find a significant difference on vowel errors between their apraxic and nonapraxic defective articulation groups. To address the issue of vowel production in children with apraxia of speech, vowel errors from the phrase imitation task were tallied. The results are presented in Table 6–6. The numerical values represent the relative strength of each vowel erred, that is the proportion of the number of times the vowel was misproduced divided by the number of times it was attempted during the speaking task. The primary vowel change was neutralization of a target to a central /ʌ/ or /ə/. In support of Morley's observations, the proportion of any vowel error was extremely low, and diphthongs were erred most frequently. It is important to remember that these data are collapsed across a group of 15 children. Obviously, some of the children made a higher proportion of vowel errors than others. This observation raises a question similar to that posed by Rosenbek and Wertz (1972). Are vowel errors diagnostically significant? Specifically, in reference to the motolinguistic model, would certain subtypes of developmental motor speech disorders (e.g., dysarthria and/or executive apraxia) be more likely to contribute to vowel production errors? Unfortunately, no published study has addressed this question.

Consonant Hierarchies and Syllable Shapes

The sound class analysis studies indicate that lingual sounds are erred more often than labial sounds, that fricative sounds are erred more than nasals and stops, that cluster errors most often result from the omission of one member of the cluster, and that, although infrequent, vowel errors are more likely to occur on attempted diphthong productions. These results seem to support the assertion by Rosenbek and Wertz (1972) that errors are related to the complexity of articulatory adjustment. The consonant error data reflect a general hierarchy: clusters > fricatives > stops > nasals; and the vowel data suggest that diphthongs are erred more than steady state vowels. Overriding these observations is the consistent finding that speech difficulties seem to be related not only to individual segments, but also to the sequential integration

Table 6–6. Proportion of vowel errors (relative strength of vowel neutralization) for 10 vowels erred in a phrase imitation task.

Vowel	Relative Strength
aɪ	.09
aʊ	.08
ɛ	.08
æ	.06
o	.04
ɔɪ	.03
e	.01
i	.01
ɪ	.01
ɔ	.01
u	.01

of these segments into various syllabic configurations. The control of syllable shapes seems to be a primary deficit in the speech produced by apraxic children. This observation raises interesting questions regarding potential relationships between phonologic deficits and limitations in other aspects of expressive language.

Phonological Limitations and Other Language Deficits

Among descriptions of children with developmental apraxia of speech there is a common tendency to mention normal receptive language abilities but deficient expressive language abilities. Aram (Aram & Nation, 1982) felt so strongly about the language component present in these children that she preferentially used the term "developmental verbal apraxia to signify that the disorder may be more comprehensive than the term *speech* implies" (p. 148). The next chapter will evaluate language performance in children with developmental motor speech disorders more closely. However, at this point, there is a study that should be mentioned because it is one of the few, if not the only study, to evaluate potential relationships among the various aspects of speech-language deficits in children demonstrating an apraxia of speech.

Potential Relationships Between Speech and Language Abilities

Crary, Landess, and Towne (1984) investigated potential relationships among 12 phonological processes, chronological age, receptive language age (as measured by a standard test), and mean length of utterance (MLU) in morphemes calculated from a conversational sample in 10 children with apraxia of speech. They concluded that low and nonsignificant correlations between MLU and chronological age or receptive language age supported the concept of an expressive language component in developmental apraxia of speech. Three phonological processes, prevocalic voicing, stopping and deletion of initial consonants, did correlate significantly with chronological age and/or receptive language age (both of which were highly correlated with each other). These processes were more prominent among the younger children in the group. More importantly, however, was the observation that no phonological process correlated significantly with expressive language ability as measured by MLU. The authors attributed this observation to the possibility that both phonologic and syntactic deficits existed in this group of children and that the two deficit areas were not related. A retrospective analysis of that study raises two relevant points. First, among all of the phonological processes, deletion of final consonants demonstrated the highest correlation with MLU. The resulting value was not impressively high ($-.42$), but, it was the highest correlation between any phonological process and MLU. The second point is that cluster reduction errors were not included in the correlation analysis. This was an oversight, especially in view of the prominence of cluster errors seen in this group of children and the significant relationships found between this phonological process and both chronological age and MLU by Crary, Welmers, and Blache (1981) in speech-language normal preschool children. For these reasons, the potential relationships were reevaluated with regression statistics to determine whether the severity ratings (relative strength) of the phonological processes, deletion of final consonants (DFC) and/or cluster reduction (CR) significantly predicted expressive language ability as measured by MLU. The results, presented in Figure 6–3, suggest that deletion of final consonants, but not cluster reduction, is related to expressive language ability as measured by MLU in the group of apraxic children studied.

These results seem to indicate a reversal of opinion from that published by Crary, Landess, and Towne (1984). This is a false impression. The original data also suggested that DFC had the strongest relationship with MLU of all phonological processes identified. The interpretation of this relationship is that high DFC values relate to lower MLU values, implying a direct relationship between phonological performance and expressive language ability. This point is potentially important for understanding developmental apraxia of speech, the differential diagnosis of developmental motor speech disorders, and designing treatment in cases of developmental apraxia of speech. At this juncture, let it suffice to imply that such a relationship is a strong possibility. More attention will be given to this matter later in this chapter and in the next chapter.

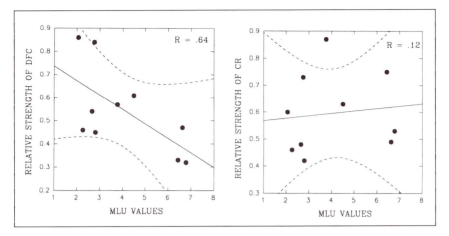

Figure 6-3. Plot of regression analyses comparing the relative strength of deletion of final consonants (left) and cluster reduction (right) to the mean length of utterance produced by 10 children with developmental apraxia of speech.

Performance Load Influences on Phonological Performance

Performance Load Influence Is Not a New Concept

One of the traditional attributes tagged to developmental motor speech disorders is that more errors are seen as the complexity of the speech task increases. Earlier, this scenario was termed the performance load factor. Complexity of articulatory adjustment might be one performance load factor (Rosenbek & Wertz, 1972), and in the preceding section on sound class analysis, this position was supported. Additional performance load factors that frequently emerge in the literature addressing developmental motor speech disorders are imitation and utterance length. Yoss and Darley (1974a) reported that more errors were observed when the number of syllables attempted increased. Chappell (1973) suggested that imitation and length factors may have diagnostic significance for developmental apraxia of speech. Aram and Glasson (1979) also implicated performance load factors, especially length of attempted utterance, as determinants of speech performance in children with an apraxia of speech. Despite all of the implications and references to the influential effects of imitation and utterance length on the speech performance of children with apraxia of speech, few objective studies have addressed the performance load issue. Bowman, Parsons, and Morris (1984) evaluated change in 25 phonological processes across six performance load combinations in seven children with an apraxia of speech. These investigators found no significant differences among performance load conditions for the average error frequency (relative strength) of the combined phonological processes. They did, however, report that two processes, deletion of final consonants and stopping, occurred more frequently in spontaneous speech than in an imitation task and that deletion of final consonants occurred more frequently in polysyllabic than in monosyllabic words. These investigators concluded that, on average, phonological errors produced by the children they studied were very consistent across performance load conditions. However, two phonological processes were negatively influenced by conditions that presumably increased the performance load of the speaking task.

Imitation and Length of Utterance

In separate studies, Ludwig and Crary (1981) and Ludwig (1983) completed extensive evaluations of the influence of performance load factors on speech patterns in children demonstrating an apraxia of speech. In the initial study (Ludwig and Crary, 1981), imitation and utterance length factors were evaluated in a group of eight children. This group produced the same 100 words under three conditions: single word repetition, phrase repetition, and in elicited conversation. Errors were subjected to a phonological process analysis. Once identified, phonological processes were categorized into two classes: syntagmatic and paradigmatic. Syntagmatic errors are those involving sound sequences. This does not necessarily mean that all syntagmatic errors are omissions. Certain types of substitution and addition errors also might be classified as syntagmatic. Paradigmatic errors are more classically identified as substitution errors that are not influenced by the sequence in which the target sound appears. Three types of analyses were completed: (1) the total number of errors within the respective speech sampling conditions, (2) the proportion of errors that were sound-sequence (syntagmatic) or sound-substitution (paradigmatic), and (3) the proportion of error types across performance load conditions (word repetition, phrase repetition, and conversation). The largest number of total errors was obtained in phrase repetition, followed by conversation and single word repetition. Statistical comparisons of these results indicated that the only significant difference was between the two repetition conditions. Significantly more errors were obtained in the phrase repetition condition. No significant differences were obtained between the phrase repetition and conversation conditions nor between the conversation and the single word repetition conditions. Although more paradigmatic than syntagmatic phonological processes were identified, the proportion of syntagmatic errors was much higher. This finding implies that errors of sound-sequence, including omission, were the dominant error type for these subjects. Finally, there seemed to be a difference in the proportion of syntagmatic, but not paradigmatic, errors across performance load conditions. Because the only significant differences were obtained between the two repetition conditions, the focus of change in the distribution of error types was between the word and phrase repetition conditions. Chi square analyses indicated that the phrase repetition condition resulted in a higher proportion of syntagmatic, but not paradigmatic, errors than the word repetition condition. In short, syntagmatic errors increased in the phrase repetition condition (higher performance load), whereas paradigmatic errors did not. Thus, not only did syntagmatic errors dominate the error profile, but only these errors were influenced by performance load factors.

Conversational Speech as a Performance Load Factor

The result that the conversation condition did not produce the greatest number of errors was not predicted by Ludwig and Crary (1981). It was presumed to be the highest performance load condition because each speaker was responsible for formulating his or her own responses versus repeating the word or phrase provided by the examiner. Also, prior reports had suggested that speech performance was most likely to be poorest in conversation. The answer to this apparent contradiction may have been found by reviewing the conversational samples. There seemed to be a tendency for the subjects to use short phrases (one, two, or three words) when attempting certain target productions. Thus conversational responses were similar in length and lexical composition to the word and phrase repetition tasks. This observation raised questions regarding the ability of these children to "trade-off" certain grammatical properties when faced with increased complexity in other properties (i.e., use a shorter utterance length when the phonological target was more complex) (Crary & Hunt, 1983). In her unpublished doctoral dissertation, Ludwig (1983) pursued the issue of performance load factors as they pertained to repetition and utterance length. In this follow-up study, however, she included procedures to control for and evaluate the influence of language variables on phonological performance.

First, in an attempt to control for the influence of the language abilities of the children in the study, Ludwig (1983) evaluated three groups of children: (1) a group of children characterized by developmental apraxia of speech, (2) a group of children matched to the apraxic group on receptive language ability, and (3) a group of children matched to the apraxic group on expressive language ability. Because the apraxic group demonstrated a receptive-expressive language split favoring receptive abilities, the receptive language matched group was the same age as the apraxic group, but the expressive language matched group was younger. Children in the apraxic and the receptive language matched groups averaged 5;7; children in the expressive language matched group averaged 4;2. The same 100 words used in the Ludwig and Crary (1981) study were employed in the word and phrase repetition conditions in this study. However, rather than try to elicit the same words in conversation, Ludwig contrived a problem solving activity designed to facilitate increased length of utterance from her subjects. She subsequently coded and grouped each resulting utterance based on the number of morphemes produced: 1 to 2 morphemes, 3 to 4, 5 to 6, or 7 and longer. Phonological process analyses were completed on all samples using the closed set of processes listed in Table 6-2. As in the prior study (Ludwig & Crary, 1981), these were subdivided into syntagmatic and paradigmatic processes. The average relative strength value for each phonological process in each performance load condition was used to identify differences among the three groups. The total number of errors also was compared among the groups for the two repetition conditions only. Finally, additional analyses were completed on the conversation samples to evaluate syllable shape control in this performance load condition. For each utterance length in conversation the proportion of attempted syllable shapes and produced syllable shapes was computed. From this rather complex study, Ludwig (1983) was able to evaluate the effects of increased utterance length both between repetition tasks and within elicited conversation.

Results from comparison of the two repetition conditions indicated that the apraxic group was different from both groups of speech-language normal children who did not differ from each other on any measure. The children with apraxia of speech, not surprisingly, made more errors than the other groups on both the single word and phrase repetition tasks. Also, the apraxic group made significantly more errors on the phrase repetition task than on the single word task. The two normal-speaking groups did not demonstrate differences between these performance load levels. Comparison of phonological processes across performance load levels indicated that only two syntagmatic processes increased between the single word and the phrase task. These were deletion of final consonants (DFC) and prevocalic voicing (PVV). Both of these changes reflect simplification of syllabic structure: DFC by reducing the number of sequential elements within the syllable and PVV by reducing the complexity of the consonant-vowel relationship.

Results from comparison of utterance lengths in the conversation condition revealed a slightly different pattern of performance. Among the 13 phonological processes evaluated across the four utterance lengths, only deletion of final consonants (DFC) revealed any influence of increased performance load. The relative strength values for DFC increased systematically with increases in utterance length. This tendency is displayed in Figure 6-4.

Unfortunately for Ludwig's hypothesis, the differences in relative strength values of final consonant deletion across utterance lengths did not reach statistical significance. In this regard, none of the 13 phonological processes studied demonstrated a statistically significant influence of increased utterance length in conversation. This was a surprising result given the apparent relationship between deletion of final consonants and performance load in the Ludwig and Crary (1981) study and in the comparison of the repetition tasks in this study. Both of these results indicated a decrease in syllabic com-

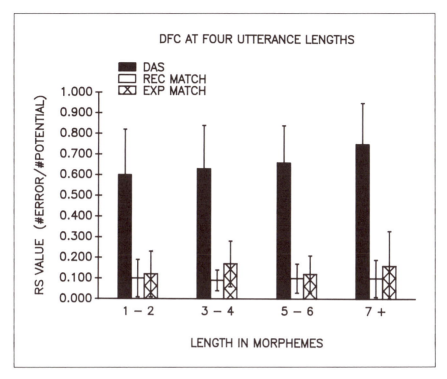

Figure 6-4. The relative strength of deletion of final consonants at four utterance lengths produced in conversation by 10 children with developmental apraxia of speech (DAS), 10 children with normal speech-language performance matched on receptive language ability (REC MATCH), and 10 children with normal speech-language performance matched on expressive language ability (EXP MATCH). (Data from Ludwig, 1983)

plexity as utterance length increased. To address this potential relationship between syllable structure control and utterance length further, Ludwig used her analysis of attempted and produced syllable shapes across the respective utterance lengths. Table 6-7 presents the proportion of attempted and produced noncluster monosyllables at the four utterance lengths. Only CV and CVC syllable shapes are included as these were the most prominent from the analyzed samples and they relate directly to syllable structure changes resulting from final consonant deletion. Attempted syllable shapes were determined from the adult form of the target word. Produced syllable shapes were identified from the child's production of each target.

These numbers lead to certain obvious conclusions. First, there seems to be little difference among the three groups with respect to the proportion of monosyllables attempted across the four utterance lengths. The only potential difference is seen as a slight increase in CVC syllable shapes in the 7 + morphemes utterances produced by the apraxic group. More important, how-

Table 6–7. Proportion of attempted and produced syllable shapes at four utterance lengths in conversation by 10 children with an apraxia of speech, 10 children matched for receptive language age and 10 children matched for expressive language ability.

	Utterance Length (in morphemes)			
Syllable Shape	1–2	3–4	5–6	7+
Apraxic Group				
CV				
Attempted	.18	.18	.30	.21
Produced	.43	.47	.42	.56
CVC				
Attempted	.39	.35	.39	.46
Produced	.18	.08	.15	.08
Receptive Language Matched Group				
CV				
Attempted	.20	.18	.21	.17
Produced	.25	.19	.24	.22
CVC				
Attempted	.32	.32	.30	.27
Produced	.29	.30	.27	.32
Expressive Language Matched Group				
CV				
Attempted	.20	.20	.17	.18
Produced	.23	.22	.21	.22
CVC				
Attempted	.35	.30	.31	.29
Produced	.32	.24	.27	.26

Source: Data from Ludwig (1983).

ever, is the obvious effect of final consonant deletion on the proportion of monosyllables produced. Little difference is noted between attempted and produced closed syllables (those ending in a consonant) in either of the two control groups. But, in the apraxic group, there is a pronounced difference at each level of utterance length. Furthermore, there seems to be an increase in the difference between the proportion of attempted and produced CVC syllables in the apraxic group as utterance length increases. However, this is not a consistent, linear trend across utterance lengths. It seems that there is sufficient fluctuation in the proportion of CVC syllables produced across the four utterance lengths to preclude any meaningful conclusion that increased utterance length in elicited conversation negatively influences control of monosyllabic forms.

Clinical Implications from Performance Load Studies

Ludwig's (Ludwig, 1983; Ludwig & Crary, 1981) series of phonological analyses raise some interesting questions that have practical, clinical significance. First, there are differences in phonological performance among children with apraxia of speech between single word and phrase repetition tasks. Ludwig's findings from both studies suggest that use of single word imitation tasks would underestimate the severity of the phonological deficit in children with an apraxia of speech. Next, when word selection is controlled (Ludwig & Crary, 1981), no significant difference in phonological performance is identified by phrase repetition versus elicited conversation tasks. Finally, when elicited conversation is used as a sampling procedure, there seems to be no consistent, negative influence of increased utterance length. This finding is the opposite of the result seen with repetition tasks. The distinction between these two results may point to inherent differences in the tasks and/or certain aspects of speech-language processing ability in these children. Ludwig (1983) implied that children with an apraxia of speech may adjust their speech-language output to accommodate their phonological limitations. Adjustments may come in the form of lexical selection based on syllable shape, altered syntactic form, and/or a simple reduction in the number of elements produced. This position is similar to what Crary and Hunt (1983) referred to as "grammatical trade-off," in which one aspect of speech-language performance was altered to accommodate another. This is a very interesting possibility which might account for absence of an utterance length effect in Ludwig's conversation condition. Unfortunately, the data do not address this issue directly. Thus, although it is possible that these children are linguistic jugglers, balancing the combined influences of phonology, lexical selection, syntactic form, and other speech-language factors, there is no proof from Ludwig's data.

There may seem to be disagreement between the results of the Bowman study (Bowman, Parsons, & Morris, 1984) and the studies completed by Ludwig. In Bowman's study, final consonant deletion was negatively influenced by increasing the performance load from imitation to spontaneous speech tasks. This result was not obtained in Ludwig's initial study. The difference in these results may be due to the fact that Ludwig controlled word selection in her conversation task. Responses in her conversation task were similar in length to the phrase repetition task. Thus, although the task environment was changed, the response characteristics (lexical selection and utterance length) remained the same. In her second study no constraints were placed on lexical selection during the conversation task. The contrast between repetition and conversation tasks in that study was similar to that used by Bowman. The results also were similar. The error frequency (relative strength) for final consonant deletion nearly doubled in the conversation task compared to either word or phrase repetition. This result agrees with both the Bowman study results and with historical perceptions of the influence of increased performance load on speech performance in children with an apraxia of speech. Perhaps the most significant observation of these studies is that sampling procedure has the potential to influence obtained results.

Subgroups of Phonological Performance

The motolinguistic model predicts different types or subgroups of developmental motor speech disorders, including different types of apraxias of speech. In Chapter 5, motor profiles from face, hand, and speech diadochokinetic performances were presented that corresponded to the predictions made by the motolinguistic model. Attempts also have been made to evaluate subgroups of developmental apraxia of speech based on phonological performance. Crary, Towne, Comeau, and Korte (1982) and Crary (1984b) described cluster analysis results on phonological process profiles from 24 children with an apraxia of speech. Simply stated, cluster analysis subdivides a group into subgroups based on similarities and differences among multiple variables. In these two studies, phonological processes were used as the distinguishing variables. Interestingly, the two analyses used different cluster analysis procedures but obtained very similar results. Three subgroups were identified: one dominated by syllable structure errors (primarily omission), one by sound-class substitution errors, and one by specific sound errors. The second analysis (Crary, 1984b) contained the more rigorous analysis procedure. In this analysis, the three groups seemed to be distinguished, not only by type of dominant phonological error, but also by the more general factor of severity. Group 1, characterized primarily by omission errors, was not the youngest group, but it did contain the most severely impaired cases. Group 2 was the youngest group, but its members were not as severely impaired as those in group 1. Group 3 members demonstrated difficulties primarily with /r/ and /l/ sounds as singletons and in clusters.

The results of these studies are not applicable to the motolinguistic model. Neither study attempted to type the subjects based on motor performance indices either before or after the cluster analysis of phonological errors. To date, no study has delineated specific types of phonological errors in children with different motor performance profiles. The results of these cluster analysis studies do, however, suggest a potential avenue of phonological alteration that occurs with overall phonological improvement. As a child's phonological ability improves, a corresponding shift in the type of dominant error would be expected. Crary (1984b) has demonstrated this pattern in a limited case example. Weckler and Crary (1982) also have reported this pattern of "phonological reorganization" in apraxic children receiving speech-language therapy.

Other Aspects of Speech Performance

Acoustic Analyses of Speech-Timing Control

Acoustic properties of speech production represent the results of activity within the vocal tract during speech. Among the many acoustic properties of speech, temporal analyses have been used to formulate inferences concerning motor control of various components within the speech mechanism. Although many acoustic analyses have been reported for both normal and disordered child speech, few, if any studies have attempted to document the acoustic properties of the speech of children with an apraxia of speech or congenital suprabulbar paresis. Glasson (1981) reported the results of spectrographic analysis of two apraxic children and indicated more acoustic irregularities in the child who demonstrated poorer speech. In a subsequent study, Glasson (1984) evaluated a variety of segment duration measures obtained from four apraxic children engaged in a sentence repetition task. The children ranged in age from 8 to 14 years. They were not thoroughly described other than to say that they met apraxic criteria and they appeared to be a heterogeneous group. Glasson's results also were heterogeneous. She observed individual differences in speech-timing control but could not conclude from these differences that her small group differed from children with normal speech-language abilities.

Voice Onset Time (VOT)

In a limited description, Crary and Towne (1984) presented voice onset time (VOT) results for five children with an apraxia of speech for labial, apical and velar prevocalic stops. Results from the apraxic group, averaging 5 years of age, were compared to data collected on the same stimulus words from normal-speaking 2- and 6-year-old children by Zlatin and Koenigsknecht (1976). Crary and Towne concluded that the children with an apraxia of speech differed from both the 2- and the 6-year-old normal speakers in several important ways. Apraxic children in this analysis did maintain acoustic distinctions between voicing categories (voiced and voiceless) for labial and velar stops, but did so with a different pattern of VOT production than was seen in the normal-speaking children. Apical stops demonstrated the least amount of timing control. This finding was interpreted as supporting Crary's (1984b) observation that apical consonants created particular difficulty for children with an apraxia of speech. The collective results of this limited analysis suggest that the children in the apraxic group did evidence limitations in the control of motor speech timing. Furthermore, the observation that voicing distinctions for two of the three places of articulation were maintained, albeit differently from either normal-speaking group of children, suggests that the children with an apraxia of speech possessed linguistic knowledge of the voicing contrast, but had to execute that knowledge in a different manner than normal-speaking children.

These limited studies indicate that children with developmental motor speech disorders demonstrate speech-timing deviations. But, more is unknown than known about these deviations. Additional studies of acoustic properties of speech segments might contribute to a better understanding of the motor control properties of children with various developmental motor speech disorders. From the motolinguistic model perspective, one would predict that different profiles of motor control would emerge from disorders at the respective ends of the continuum.

Prosodic Deviations in Speech Production

In simple terms, prosody refers to the melody of speech. Prosodic features of speech may signal linguistic (i.e., statement versus question) or emotional information. There is no single prosodic attribute of speech. Stress, intonation, and timing characteristics of speech segments, at times referred to as suprasegmental, are often considered key prosodic features. Given the basic nature of dysarthrias, clinicians would expect prosodic deviations in dysarthric speech. Darley, Aronson, and Brown (1975) described many prosodic deviations in several different dysarthrias in adults. Unfortunately, due to the paucity of clinical and research information surrounding the developmental dysarthria associated with congenital suprabulbar paresis, little is known about prosodic deviations in this developmental motor speech disorder. The scenario is not much different for developmental apraxia of speech. Although many authors have referred to prosodic disturbances in this developmental motor speech disorder, no published study has specifically addressed prosodic deviations in children with developmental apraxia of speech.

Rosenbek and Wertz (1972) described several prosodic deviations among children with apraxia of speech. These included slower rate, equalized stress, and syllabic segregation. These observations would characterize the child with an apraxia of speech as a slow speaker, with nearly the same stress pattern on each syllable and with notable pauses between syllables. Yoss and Darley (1974a) also commented on slow rate and equalized stress patterns, especially among older children. Aram and Glasson (1979) reported impressions parallel to those of Yoss and Darley. In one of the few studies attempting to evaluate prosodic characteristics of children with apraxia of speech, Tallman and Crary (1985) compared seven children with developmental apraxia of speech to seven children with normal speech-language performance matched for age and receptive language ability. Their task involved an imitation procedure in which all subjects repeated three word sentences. The prosodic features were chosen so that half of the sentences were perceived as statements and the other half were perceived as questions. Based on acoustic analyses of the imitated sentences, Tallman and Crary (1985) concluded that the children in the apraxic group did not confuse the linguistic aspects of prosody in their responses, but that they were less efficient than speech-language normal group in producing the prosodic distinctions. Figure 6–5 presents average responses for the production of statements versus questions by the respective groups. The intonation (fundamental frequency) and temporal (timing/duration) characteristics of the averaged responses are displayed.

Many of the acoustic findings in this study support prior clinical impressions offered by Rosenbek and Wertz and others. The primary prosodic differences between the apraxic and the speech-language normal groups were: less intonation variation (reduced sentence intonation slope and reduced range and slope of the terminal contour of questions), longer sentence durations, and longer intersyllabic pauses. Average fundamental frequency and fundamental frequency range across each response did not differ between the two groups. Syllable durations did not differ with the exception of the third syllable which was actually shorter in the apraxic group. These acoustic results may well contribute to the perception of slower rate, equalized stress, and syllabic segregation in the speech of children with an apraxia of speech. To address this issue more completely, additional research needs to be conducted. From the motolinguistic model perspective, differences would be expected between individuals at the executive (dysarthria and executive apraxia) and the planning ends of the continuum. Children at the executive end of the continuum might be expected to have more severe prosodic deviations than those at the planning end, if for no other reason than the potential for more severe deficits in motor speech control.

Summary Comments: Unanswered Questions

A nagging complaint concerning speech performance in the child with a developmental motor speech disorder is whether characteristics of speech performance are diagnostic of that particular disorder. The response to this complaint might be "sometimes yes and sometimes no." Among children with dysarthria certain speech abnormalities may relate directly to underlying motor deficits. Unfortunately, the relationship between speech errors and motor control properties in the child with an apraxia of speech is much cloudier (like the Florida Keys during a thunderstorm). It would be erroneous to assume that every child who omits a final consonant demonstrates an apraxia of speech, or that children who do not omit consonants are not apraxic. Some speech performance characteristics, however, do seem to indicate the possibility of an apraxia of speech: multiple errors dominated by omissions, negative influence of increased performance load, dysprosody, and perhaps other more microscopic clues identified via acoustic analyses. Perhaps with additional research, we will begin to understand the potential relationships be-

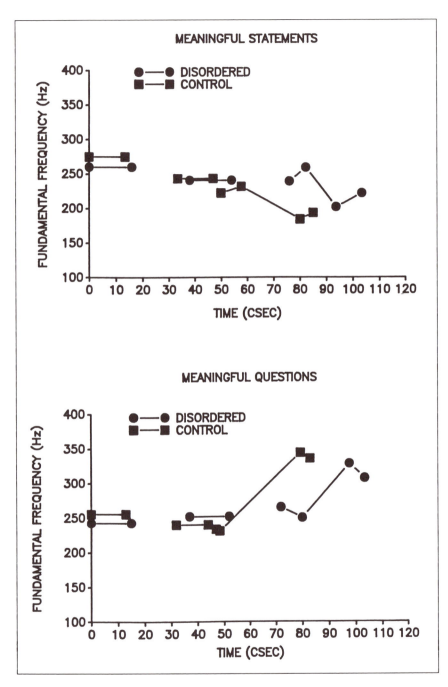

Figure 6–5. Comparison of prosodic contours of statements (top) and questions (bottom) produced by children with developmental apraxia of speech (disordered) versus children with normal speech-language abilities. (Data from Tallman & Crary, 1985)

tween various motor control profiles and specific speech performance profiles. At the present time, however, we will do well to remember that developmental apraxias of speech are better identified by motor symptoms and patterns of motor speech performance than by specific speech production errors.

Think About This

Developmental motor speech disorders are characterized by severe and persistent speech production deficits. However, no available information supports the assertion that the various developmental motor speech disorders are identified by specific speech performance patterns. Many reports do, however, agree on general speech performance attributes relative to dysarthria or apraxia of speech. Among the more salient observations are the following:

1. The dysarthria seen in the incomplete form of congenital suprabulbar paresis is expected to be characterized by specific sound error patterns related to the anatomy of the spastic weakness. A similar expectation exists for the complete syndrome but with the consideration that multiple aspects of the speech mechanism may be involved creating a more widespread disturbance to the developing sound system.

2. Children with an apraxia of speech are expected to demonstrate a multitude of speech errors of varying types. They differ both quantitatively and qualitatively from children with normal speech-language performance.

3. When considering groups of children, the dominant speech errors in developmental apraxias of speech are errors of omission involving both single consonants and clusters. Expect variations to this observation.

4. Increased performance load is expected to have a negative influence on the speech performance of the child with an apraxia of speech. Its influence on the speech of children with dysarthria is unknown.

5. Many children with a developmental apraxia of speech will demonstrate prosodic deviations including slowed rate, equalized stress, and prolonged pauses between words and syllables.

6. Subgroups of speech performance may exist, but these have not been related to the motor performance profiles depicted by the motolinguistic model.

7. **Available evidence suggests that speech performances of children with a developmental motor speech disorder are differentially influenced by evaluation techniques.**

Depending on the purpose for which these observations are used, they may be either a blessing or a curse. It would seem inappropriate to use specific speech patterns to differentially diagnose a developmental motor speech disorder from any other developmental communication deficit or to separate the various developmental motor speech disorders. The information available is insufficient. However, these observations may be helpful as general guiding principles from which to ask further empirical questions about developmental motor speech disorders or to plan the evaluation of speech performance in such cases.

CHAPTER
Seven

Language Performance

Language Performance in Dysarthric Children

A Matter of Percentages

The primary emphasis in developmental motor speech disorders has been, for good reason, on poor speech performance. However, as presented in Chapter 1, there are frequent references to impaired language performance among children with developmental motor speech disorders. Morley, Court, and Miller (1954) reported that 50% of the children they studied with developmental dysarthria (including articulatory apraxia) demonstrated associated disorders of language. Related language disorders included dyslexia, dysgraphia, delayed onset of speech, and/or limited vocabulary. The extent of these language deficits varied widely among the children studied. In a subsequent paper, Morley, Court, Miller, and Garside (1955) stated that, although dysarthria and aphasia (here defined as the internal comprehension and formulation of words) may coexist in the same child, the two bear no intrinsic relationship. Worster-Drought (1974) reported that approximately 30% (62 of 200) of the children he studied with congenital suprabulbar paresis demonstrated some form of spoken language deficit in addition to defective articulation. The vast majority of these children demonstrated expressive language deficits. The general position of these early authors seems to be that language deficits may coexist with developmental dysarthria in some children; however, the two disorders are not intrinsically related. Language deficits in dysarthric children vary widely in type and severity, especially if delayed speech onset and written language difficulties are included among the language limitations. When focusing solely on spoken language deficits, the primary pattern seems to be limitations in expressive language performance with spared or comparatively superior receptive language performance.

Language Performance in Apraxia of Speech

Family Members Or Near Neighbors

A similar, but slightly different, picture is painted for children with apraxia of speech. Morley, Court, Miller, and Garside (1955) felt that articulatory apraxia was related to developmental aphasia, specifically expressive aphasia. However, because their experiences included several children who demonstrated apraxia of speech without impairment in the development of language, they concluded that, although these two disorders were near neighbors, they were separate entities. When these entities do coexist in the same child, the aphasia, or language deficit, is more likely to be in expressive aspects of language performance.

Since these early observations little attention has been given to the language abilities of children with developmental motor speech disorders. Rosenbek and Wertz (1972) reported that 40% (20 of 50) of the apraxic children they studied demonstrated a concomitant apraxia and aphasia. An additional 16% (8 of 50) demonstrated concomitant apraxia, dysarthria, and aphasia. In this respect, over half of the children they studied demonstrated a concomitant aphasia and developmental motor speech disorder. Rosenbek and Wertz suggested that the incidence of aphasia might have been higher in their subjects, but limitations of their study and disagreement of what constitutes developmental aphasia precluded a more detailed analysis. These authors also concluded that receptive abilities are inordinately superior to expressive language abilities, especially in children who are free of language deficits. The qualifier to their statement introduces confusion into the clinical picture. Perhaps, Rosenbek and Wertz were referring to aphasia as a primary receptive language deficit and implying that, even in nonaphasic children, an expressive language deficit was observed. Despite this confusion, the conclusion from this report—that apraxia may coexist with language deficits and receptive language abilities are superior to expressive language abilities—has influenced many studies of developmental apraxia of speech. One implication from these observations and conclusions is that apraxia of speech and language deficits (aphasia) are distinct clinical entities that may coexist.

Keeping Language Deficits Separate

Yoss and Darley (1974a) did not study language performance in children with apraxia of speech but did influence the perception of language abilities in these children by setting language criteria in their selection of subjects.

These investigators specified that all of the children in their study demonstrated a language development age within 6 months of their chronological age. To determine language performance Yoss and Darley employed the *Utah Test of Language Development* (Mecham, Jex, & Jones, 1967). This test evaluates rather general aspects of language performance and provides a single language development age score. In this respect, it is not possible even to infer potential differences between receptive and expressive language performance. Aram (Aram & Nation, 1982) has criticized the use of this test to qualify children as language normal due to its general nature and the absence of syntactic analyses. Thus , there may have been language deficits among Yoss and Darley's subjects that were not delineated by the language test they used. Nonetheless, the decision by Yoss and Darley to exclude children with more overt language deficits is not without ramifications. One implication is that these investigators felt that apraxia of speech was distinct from language deficits. This position would be in agreement with prior historical perspective. Another implication is that Yoss and Darley simply wanted to control for possible sources of variation in their data. Including children who had language deficits might well have obscured the purpose of their study as well as changed their results. Again, the implication is that language deficits are not central to developmental apraxia of speech. The reality of the situation is that these investigators used a rather general language test to exclude children with language deficits from their study of developmental apraxia of speech. Limitations of the language test used do not preclude the possibility that some of the children in their study had language performance deficits in addition to speech performance deficits.

An Island on the Sea of Motor Speech Separatists

Aram's (Aram & Nation, 1982) position concerning language performance in children with apraxia of speech seems much like an island on a sea of motor speech separatists. She felt that the inherent deficits in developmental apraxia of speech involved more than just speech production. In a series of studies she detailed language performance in eight children who demonstrated apraxia of speech. Aram's intent was to control potential confounding variables toward the goal of understanding language abilities in children with apraxia of speech. For this reason she included only those children who demonstrated normal nonverbal intelligence, normal language comprehension (at least on some tasks), had normal hearing, and demonstrated no evidence of dysarthria but demonstrated persistent articulation disorders that were slow to respond to speech therapy. Language development milestones (see Chapter 4), language comprehension, language formulation, and accompanying learning disabilities were evaluated in each of her eight subjects. Her initial findings (Aram & Nation, 1982) included:

1. Comprehension of semantics and syntax are often normal, if nonverbal mental age is normal.
2. Length of sentences negatively affects sentence comprehension.
3. Limitations in semantic formulation, ranging from mild to severe, are usually present.
4. Formulated syntax is disordered, presenting deficiencies in inflectional markers as well as selection and sequencing of syntactic elements.
5. Reading, writing, and spelling difficulties are typically apparent at school age. (pp. 160–161)

These findings led Aram (Aram & Nation, 1982) to conclude that "developmental verbal apraxia is not confined to the phonologic and articulatory aspects of speech. Rather, all levels of formulated language may be affected, including the lexical, syntactic, and phonologic aspects" (p. 161).

There are at least three ways to consider this conclusion. One way is to accept that language deficits often accompany developmental motor speech disorders without any consideration of the relationship between the two areas of performance. This position should produce little controversy because it is a common description in most reports on dysarthria and apraxia of speech in children. A second position would be a literal interpretation of Aram's conclusion: Language deficits are an integral part of developmental apraxia of speech (developmental verbal apraxia). This view portrays an underlying information processing deficit common to both speech and language functions. This position may contribute to controversy because it deviates from tradition by including language processing deficits within a motor speech disorder. Most prior reports attempted to separate speech and language factors in describing developmental motor speech disorders. A third position would be that speech and language processing deficits coexist such that deficits in one aspect (speech) contribute to the other (language). The motolinguistic model would predict that in certain types of motor speech disorders (i.e., planning variants of apraxia of speech), language processing deficits are more probable (Chapter 3). In other types of motor speech deficits (i.e., dysarthria and executive variants of apraxia of speech), language performance deficits may be the result of speech limitations. The suggestion is that different types of language deficits might be encountered in different forms of developmental motor speech disorders. Unfortunately, no substantial body of information is available that allows us to address this issue with any degree of wisdom. Likewise, there is a poor understanding of the underlying processing deficits that contribute to limitations in language performance among children with developmental motor speech disorders. These distinctions may be important for clinicians addressing concomitant speech and language problems in children with developmental motor speech disorders. Therefore a more detailed look at Aram's initial findings may serve as a starting point toward a better understanding of potential relationships between speech and language processes in developmental motor speech disorders.

Language Comprehension

Performance Load Factors in Comprehension: Length of Input

Aram (Aram & Nation, 1982) reported that language comprehension is often normal if nonverbal intelligence is normal. This is a statement rather than a conclusion because Aram, like many other investigators, selected subjects based partly on age-appropriate language comprehension abilities. However, her conclusion that language comprehension is negatively influenced by length of sentences is very interesting. This conclusion is based on performances on different comprehension tests: *Assessment of Children's Comprehension of Language* (ACLC) (Foster, Giddan, & Stark, 1972); *Northwestern Syntax Screening Text* (NSST) (Lee, 1969), and *The Token Test for Children* (DiSimoni, 1978). Each of these procedures claims to vary length and complexity of language comprehension stimuli. But, these procedures are not equivalent, and none of Aram's subjects completed all three. Therefore, any conclusion regarding language comprehension processing deficits drawn from that analysis is based on limited, unequal comprehension assessment procedures. Table 7–1 presents the results of language comprehension testing completed by Aram (Aram & Nation, 1982).

A score within normal limits on the NSST may be used to demonstrate appropriate comprehension of syntactic elements of spoken language as measured by this test. Without a more detailed analysis of individual NSST items, however, the score from this procedure cannot be used to substantiate Aram's conclusion that increased length of sentences negatively influences comprehension. In this regard, the single child (JP) whose only comprehension score was a 50th percentile score on the NSST might be eliminated from consideration on the length influence issue. The ACLC systematically increases the length of stimuli from two to three to four comprehension elements. Data from four of the eight children are presented for this task. Of these four children, two (SC and JK) made no comprehension errors across the various levels of the ACLC, while two (AS and JS) demonstrated the described deterioration in performance as item length increased. A stronger argument for this position might be made from the Token Test data. This procedure systematically increases length of stimuli over four levels with a final level focused on syntactic comprehension rather than stimulus length. Four children completed this protocol, with complete data being presented for three of the four (no data were presented for level IV for subject MN). If length of stimuli was the critical factor then the performance pattern should reveal a deterioration in

Table 7–1. Comprehension of connected speech in eight children with developmental verbal apraxia.

Child	ACLC (% Correct)			NSST (percentile)	Token Test (SD)				
	2 Elements	3 Elements	4 Elements		I	II	III	IV	V
JP				50th					
AS	90/93.2	60/74.9	70/63.4						
MN				>50th	OK	OK	−1SD		+1SD
JS	90/94.3	80/90.1	40/83.6						
SC	100%	100%	100%						
PB				30/40	OK	OK	OK	−2SD	−1SD
PO					OK	OK	−2SD	−3SD	−1SD
JK	100%	100%	100%		OK	OK	−1SD	−1SD	−3SD

Source: From Aram, D., and Nation, J. (1982). *Child language disorders* (p. 158). St. Louis: C.V. Mosby. Reprinted by permission.

performance from levels I to IV of this test with a recovery of performance in level V (where the focus is on syntactic complexity rather than length). This pattern is only partially demonstrated in the data. One subject (PO) demonstrated the expected pattern while two others (MN and PB) demonstrated "close enough" performance profiles. The fourth subject (JK), who incidentally made no errors on the ACLC, produced the poorest performance on the final, syntactic subtest. In short, although there is some individual data to support the claim that language comprehension is adversely influenced by length of input, the published data do not uniformly support this claim as a conclusion pertaining to all children demonstrating apraxia of speech. However, there may be other, closely related reasons for observed variation in language comprehension abilities.

Information Processing and Resource Allocation

In Chapter 2, McNeil's position on resource allocation (McNeil, Odell, & Tseng, 1991) was discussed. Information processed appropriately in one cognitive environment may be processed inappropriately in a more demanding cognitive environment. Length of information may be a factor in changing the cognitive environment even when other potential factors are consistent. An example of this is seen in the performance load studies of phonological performance discussed in Chapter 6. In the comprehension data presented by Aram (Table 7–1), length may have been a factor for some children, but not for all. For some children (i.e., JK), the additional factor of increased syntactic complexity combined with length may have been required to impair comprehension performance. In others, length, syntactic complexity, attention, and/or other factors combined were insufficient to detract from the comprehension performance. A common denominator seems to be that some of these children do demonstrate limitations in information processing that may influence language comprehension abilities. Based on present knowledge, it would be premature to specify any individual factor as a primary negative influence in the comprehension performance in all children with developmental motor speech disorders.

Language Formulation

Expressive Deficits: What Did You Say?

Claims that children with developmental motor speech disorders demonstrate limitations in the expressive aspects of spoken language should not be surprising. In many, if not most cases, speech production is so poor that little of what is said is understood by the listener. Most reports specify that such children demonstrate a "receptive-expressive split" in language performance with poorer expressive language abilities. A key issue in this respect is not the presence of expressive language deficits, but rather the nature of expressive language deficits. This distinction is important for understanding language formulation deficits and for intervening in individual cases. Aram (Aram & Nation, 1982) contended that children with apraxia of speech demonstrate both semantic and syntactic formulation deficits. The semantic formulation deficits she identified revolve around lexical selection and use. They apparently were not present in every child and may have been more prominent among the younger children. Aram's conclusions (Aram and Nation, 1982) included:

1. No child demonstrated a normal expressive vocabulary. Deficits ranged from mild to severe.
2. Several younger children used gestures and onomatopoeic sounds to convey intended meaning.
3. Two of the younger children used almost no verb forms.
4. Most of the children had difficulty with prepositions.
5. Several of the children were anomic, often using related words.

Semantic Formulation Deficits: Mean What You Say and Say What You Mean

It is difficult to interpret Aram's observations in specific reference to developmental motor speech disorders. The presence of semantic formulation limitations in some children, predominantly younger children, does not prove that children with apraxia of speech uniformly demonstrate such deficits. From a neurolinguistic perspective, semantic deficits might be associated more with posterior hemisphere dysfunction (see Chapter 2). In this respect, the motolinguistic model would predict that such limitations would be more prevalent among children with a planning variant of apraxia of speech. Another more obvious consideration exists, however. Is it possible that these semantic formulation deficits might be related to a language system developing out of balance? Or to attempts by the child to compensate for limitations in information processing by manipulating those aspects of speech-language over which he or she does have some degree of control? Both of these alternatives might explain the presence of lexical errors in the speech of apraxic children; neither would implicate semantic deficits as a cause of these alterations. Semantic formulation deficits in the form of lexical selection and use errors may be seen in children with developmental motor speech disorders, and clinicians are encouraged to include these types of analyses in the evaluation; however, insufficient information is available to conclude that semantic formulation deficits are a necessary component of developmental apraxia of speech.

Syntactic Deficits: Short But Not Sweet

Deficits in syntactic formulation also would be expected among children with expressive language limitations. And, as previously stated, expressive language limitations are the dominant language deficit among children with motor speech disorders. In Aram's initial study of syntactic formulation deficits in children with apraxia of speech, she compared *Developmental Sentence Scores* (Lee, 1974) from six apraxic children to the 50th percentile score for each child's age. Two of the six children were omitted from this comparison because they demonstrated only rudimentary syntactic abilities. Results of this comparison supported prior assertions of expressive language deficits. Each of the apraxic children scored well below the 50th percentile for his or her age. Aram (Aram & Nation, 1982) commented that, "although these children had difficulty with inflectional endings, they also had notable difficulty with word order, pronoun number and case, use of clauses, and so forth" (p. 159).

Ekelman and Aram (1983) recognized the limitations of a single score to describe syntactic formulation deficits and completed a more comprehensive analysis of expressive language (syntactic) performance in spontaneous speech from eight children with apraxia of speech. They utilized four measures to indicate various aspects of syntactic complexity: mean length of utterance (MLU) used to establish Brown's five developmental language stages (Brown, 1973), *Developmental Sentence Score* (Lee, 1974), analyses of 14 grammatical markers (de Villiers & de Villiers, 1973; Miller, 1981), and analyses of yes-no and wh-questions (Miller, 1981). Ekelman and Aram identified the presence of many syntactic errors, even in children whose MLU values placed them above Brown's stage V of grammatical development. Table 7-2 summarizes their findings.

On average, their subjects demonstrated syntactic errors on just over 50% of their attempted sentences. Additionally, there seemed to be substantial var-

Table 7-2. Summary of syntactic deficits observed in the spontaneous speech of eight children with developmental apraxia of speech studied by Ekelman and Aram (1983).

1. Pronoun errors

2. Complete verb omissions

3. Omission and/or incorrect use of many grammatical markers, especially at and beyond stage V of syntactic development

4. Auxiliary and/or copula omission in yes-no and wh-questions

5. Auxiliary and/or copula not inverted in yes-no and wh-questions

6. Incorrect auxiliary substitutions

7. Omission of do support in yes-no and wh-questions

iability in the expression of a variety of grammatic structures among the eight subjects. Across each of the syntactic analyses, omission errors dominated. There were instances of substitution errors and word order errors, but these seemed much less frequent than omission errors. Based on their analyses, Ekelman and Aram (1983) concluded that "at least some of the errors presented by this group of apraxic children cannot be attributed to motor speech and/or phonologic limitations but rather evidence concomitant syntactic disorders" (p. 250). This assertion may be correct, but, there are at least two points to consider. First, it seems apparent that some of the syntactic errors observed in children with an apraxia of speech are not the *direct* result of motor speech and/or phonologic limitations. Omissions of inflectional endings or even complete words might be attributable directly to motor speech limitations. Certain substitution errors or errors of word order, however, do not lend themselves easily to a direct motor speech limitation explanation. This does not exclude an indirect relationship. The same alternative explanations offered in reference to semantic formulation deficits may be applied here. Syntactic errors imply a simplification of the grammar at some level of language processing. The question is "which level?" Ekelman and Aram emphasized that their results were consistent with a disordered expressive language system (i.e., one that has developed abnormally rather than just slower than expected). The question might be posed (again): "Might some, if not most, of the observed syntactic errors reflect either abnormal learning or compensation on the part of the developing child to adjust for the interference of another, related problem?" The presence of appropriate language comprehension abilities in these children implies that they had knowledge of at least some of the syntactic structures that they erred in production. An interference effect seems as plausible an explanation as a common or even concomitant processing deficit explanation. A second, not necessarily unrelated point to consider is the apparent dominance of omission errors. It is not possible to confirm that omission errors were the dominant error type, given the procedures used in that study. However, omission errors certainly figured prominently among all grammatical analyses reported. If this assumption is correct and errors of omission are the direct result of motor speech and/or phonologic limitations, then Ekelman and Aram's conclusion would change to "most of the syntactic errors found in apraxic children appear to be the direct result of influences from motor speech and/or phonologic limitations." This is an important clinical consideration. Yet, as with many aspects of developmental motor speech disorders, there are only a few reports that pertain directly to this question.

Running Interference: The Role of Morphophonemic Errors

Recall from Chapter 6, the proposed relationship between MLU and deletion of final consonants. This inverse relationship implied that children who delete many final consonants have lower mean length of utterance values. One explanation of this finding is that the omitted components of language shorten the average length of utterance. That is to say that phonological limitations directly influence grammatical performance. Ekelman and Aram (1983) identified syntactic errors that apparently are not related directly to motor speech and/or phonologic limitations. However, the majority of syntactic errors identified by these investigators seem to have been omissions, including omitted final consonants. One issue raised by this observation is the proportion of syntactic errors directly attributable to phonologic simplification versus nonphonologically motivated syntactic errors. Comeau and Crary (1982) investigated this question by evaluating the percent of morphophonemic errors in the conversational speech of 14 children with an apraxia of speech. The children ranged in age from 3 to 13 years with an average age of 6 years 4 months (just over 2 years younger than the children studied by Ekelman and Aram). Fifty utterances from recorded conversation were transcribed phonetically and analyzed for the presence of two types of grammatical errors: morphophonemic and nonmorphophonemic. Morphophonemic errors were the result of a phonological error that created an omission of a bound morpheme in obligatory context. If the resultant production was phonologically incorrect but grammatically correct, the item was not counted as an error. An example of this situation is the production of /d ɔ z/for /d ɔ gz/. Because the grammatical morpheme was present, the item was scored as correct. Nonmorphophonemic errors resulted from a syntactic change that was not related to phonological simplification. Using a combination of Brown's (1973) 14 grammatical morphemes and Miller's (1981) sentence analysis procedures, 19 possible error types were identified. Six errors were considered morphophonemic or phonologically motivated, and 13 errors were considered nonmorphophonemic or nonphonologically motivated. These are listed in Table 7–3.

Error percentages were computed by calculating the number of occurrences of a given error divided by the potential occurrences of that error from the sample. For comparison purposes, data from the apraxic group were compared to data obtained from 14 children with normal speech-language abilities between 3 and 4 years of age (average age 3 years, 10 months). Figure 7–1 presents the performances of the two groups of children. An important point to consider is that the apraxic group demonstrated syntactic errors on an average of 22% of the syntactic constructions analyzed with a range from 4% to 36%. Thus, these children were more often syntactically correct than incorrect. As seen in Figure 7–1, when syntactic errors were made by the children in the apraxic group, they were primarily the result of phonological simplification. An average of 86% of the syntactic errors from the apraxic group were the result of phonological simplification. Six of the 14 children in this group demonstrated 100% of their syntactic errors in this category. In fact, only two of the children with an apraxia of speech demonstrated less than 70% phonologically motivated syntactic errors (8% and 9%, respectively). And, even in

Table 7-3. Phonologically (morphophonemic) and nonphonologically (nonmorphophonemic) motivated syntactic error types evaluated in the conversational speech of children with developmental apraxia of speech and speech-language normal children.

Phonologically Motivated Error Types			
Grammatical Morphemes	Phonological Form	Orthography	Example
1. Regular Plurals	/dɔgz/	dogs	Two dogs
2. Regular Present Third Person Singular	/rʌnz/	runs	He runs.
3. Possessives	/bɔɪz/	boy's	The boy's bike.
4. Past Regular	/lʊkt/	looked	He looked
5. Contracted Copula	/ɪts/	it's	It's red.
6. Contracted Auxiliary	/hiz/	he's	He's fast.

Nonphonologically Motivated Error Types	
Syntactic Morpheme	Example
1. Present Progressive	The boy is run*ning*.
2. Prepositions	The key is *in* my pocket.
3. Articles	I want *the* book.
4. Uncontractible Auxiliary	This *is* going up.
5. Uncontractible Copula	*Is* it wet?
6. Irregular Past Tense	The big tree *fell*.
7. Irregular Third Person Singular	He *has* a ball.
8. Pronouns	*She* wants to sing.
9. Negation	I'm *not* going.
10. Yes-No Questions	*Is it* big?
11. Wh-Questions	*Where* am I?
12. Compound Marking	I want it *but* he won't give it to me.
13. Clause Markers	We can't play *when* it rains.

Source: Adapted from Crary and Comeau (1982)

these cases, there was a higher percentage of phonologically motivated errors than nonphonologically motivated errors (2% and 6%, respectively). No child in the speech-language normal group demonstrated more than 16% phonologically motivated syntactic errors. Conversely, there was no difference between the two groups for the percentage of nonphonologically motivated syntactic errors. The apraxic group averaged 12% errors in this category compared to 9% in the speech-language normal group. These data strongly suggest that the vast majority of syntactic errors in the conversational speech of the child apraxic speakers studied were the direct result of phonological simplification.

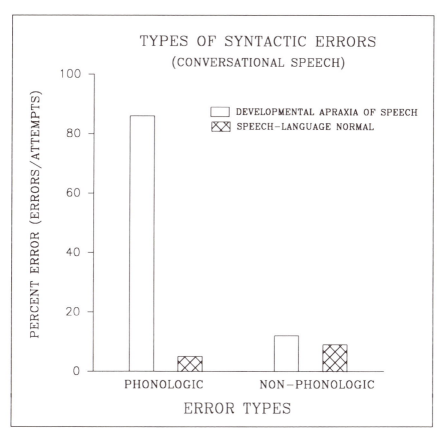

Figure 7–1. Distribution of phonologically versus nonphonologically motivated syntactic errors in the conversational speech of children with apraxia of speech versus children with normal speech-language abilities. (Data from Comeau & Crary, 1982)

The Importance of Syllable Shape

A secondary analysis in this study (Comeau & Crary, 1982) evaluated the influence of syllable shape on the application of morphophonemic rules and the influence of morphophonemic rules on syllable closure in children with apraxia of speech. This assessment was completed by computing the distribution of syllable shapes in instances when morphophonemic rules (phonologically motivated category) were produced versus when they were not produced. Remember that a rule could be applied without correct phonological production of the target word. Table 7–4 presents the results of this analysis in reference to the percentage of morphophonemic rule applications and the distribution of resulting syllable shapes produced when the rules were applied versus not applied.

The division of rule application was nearly identical in both syllable shape categories (CVC and CVCC). Morphophonemic rules were nearly three times

Table 7–4. Distribution of morphophonemic rule application relative to syllable shape.

Target Syllable Shape	Rule Applied (%)	Rule Not Applied (%)
CVC	28	72
Produced Syllables		
CVC	28	–
CV	–	72
CVCC	24	76
Produced Syllables		
CVCC	9	–
CVC	15	18
CV	–	58

Source: Adapted from Comeau and Crary (1982).

as likely *not* to be applied in both cases. Although this group of children deleted an average of 50% of final consonants, they applied morphophonemic rules only about 25% of the time. These findings suggest that the presence of a morphophonemic rule has little positive influence on the accuracy of the produced syllable shape in either CVC or CVCC targets and may have a negative influence. Consider the distribution of CVCC productions. Thirty-three percent of the resultant productions were CVC syllables. Of these, 15% incorporated the morphophonemic rule while 18% did not. One interpretation of these data is that the context of a morphophonemic rule does not increase the possibility of syllable closure. A second inference to be made from these results is that some degree of control over syllable shape is important to the development of morphophonemic rule application. The high percentage of phonologically motivated errors and the high proportion of open syllables in instances requiring morphophonemic rule application would seem to support this contention. A relevant clinical implication of these observations is the concept of bottom-up interference.

Bottom-Up Interference

The basic tenets of bottom-up interference in reference to developmental motor speech disorders have been stated or implied throughout the earlier chapters of this book. Bottom-up interference implies that deficits at the bottom of a behavior hierarchy will contribute to deficits at higher levels within that hierarchy, that is, interference works from the bottom up. Implications for developmental motor speech disorders include the position that sensorimotor deficits contribute to disordered phonological development and that phonological deficits contribute to disordered expressive language development. Children with developmental motor disorders more often than not demonstrate sensorimotor, phonological, and grammatical deficits. Although each of these should be included in a comprehensive evaluation of the child with a developmental motor speech disorder, attempts should be made to evaluate potential interactions among these respective components of motor speech disorders. At times the interactions may emerge in surprising ways. Consider the case described by Crary (1984a) of an apraxic child whose fricative errors accounted for over half of all of his phonologic errors. Evaluation of syntactic performance indicated many errors on constructions requiring fricative productions. The same syntactic constructions were correctly expressed in contexts not requiring fricative production. Crary (1984a) indicated this to be an example of bottom-up interference in the expressive grammar. The child obviously had linguistic knowledge of the various syntactic rules, but was unable to express those rules in demanding contexts—in this case, those requiring fricative productions. Brief examples of this pattern are presented in Table 7–5.

Observations like this fricative-induced agrammatism or bottom-up interference in general may be a reflection of performance-based processing deficits. This would be compatible with the performance load constraints described in Chapter 6 and with McNeil's resource allocation theory described in Chapter 2. It is possible that children with developmental motor speech disorders possess more linguistic knowledge (phonologic, semantic, syntactic) than their overt performances would indicate. The expression of this knowledge may be determined, at least in part, by a variety of factors constraining the productive use of linguistic information. Although this theoretical position may be considered as so much fodder for future research, clinicians would do well to include evaluation of potential interactions between phonological performance and expressive language performance in their assessment of children with developmental motor speech disorders.

Table 7–5. Examples of bottom-up interference in expressive language performance, in this instance, deficit fricative production contributing to syntactic errors.

Syntactic Form	Target Production	Incorrect	Correct
Auxiliary + progressive verb	She is reading.	/hʒ widin/	
	They are riding.		/deɪ ar waɪdin/
Subjective pronoun	she	/hʒ/	
	We, he		/wi, hi/
Irregular past tense	saw	/ki/	
	caught		/kɔt/

Source: Adapted from Crary (1984a).

Summary Comments: So Much To Do, So Little To Work With

Precious little systematic work has been directed at language ability among children with developmental motor speech disorders. Still, many children with developmental motor speech disorders demonstrate deficient language abilities. For the most part, these deficits are in the realm of expressive language performance with receptive language performance being normal or near-normal and superior to expressive language. This scenario is predicated on normal or near-normal intelligence. Questions arise over the nature of expressive language deficits that pertain specifically to developmental apraxia of speech. Most authors have indicated that apraxia of speech and expressive language deficits are concomitant disorders (i.e., they coexist with little or no intrinsic relationship). Although reaching different conclusions, the work of Aram and Crary deviates from this position. Aram has offered the view that language deficits are part of the information processing deficit seen in apraxic children, that is, she believes that apraxia of speech encompasses more than just defective speech processes. Crary has indicated that many expressive language deficits may be the direct result of phonological simplification and that others may be the indirect result of the same information processing deficits seen in such children. The motolinguistic model does not directly address language performance. The model suggests that children at the planning end of the continuum would be more likely to demonstrate language processing problems. One implication, based on neurolinguistic principles reviewed in Chapter 2, is that these language problems would incorporate semantic and syntactic as well as phonologic aspects. Also, presumably because the planning end of the continuum is approaching the posterior left hemisphere language areas, language abilities would be more suspect in planning variants of the disorder. The model implies that children at the opposite ends of the continuum will demonstrate different language profiles. In any given child demonstrating any variant of a developmental motor speech disorder, one or more of the language deficits described in this chapter may be present. Clinicians would be in grave error to focus exclusively on speech production characteristics in children with developmental motor speech disorders ignoring other aspects of communicative performance.

Think About This

Despite a paucity of knowledge specific to the languge abilities of children with developmental motor speech disorders, certain observations have persisted for nearly 40 years. In some cases there is agreement on the type of language deficit, but disagreement on the underlying cause. As in the case of speech performance, it would be inappropriate to use a specific language perform-ance profile to delineate a specific developmental motor speech disorder. However, historically persistent observations may serve as clinically useful guidelines for evaluation and treatment. Some of these observations include:

1. In most cases, receptive language abilities will be normal and/or superior to expressive language abilities.

2. Although semantic formulation deficits may be present, the dominant ex-pressive errors typically involve syntactic formulation.

3. The majority of syntactic errors appear to result from limitations in pho-nological performance, and interactions between phonological and syn-tactic performances suggest the operation of a bottom-up interference in the expressive grammar.

4. **Evaluation and intervention strategies in cases of developmental motor speech disorders should include description of language abil-ities and consideration of the potential interaction between speech and language performance.**

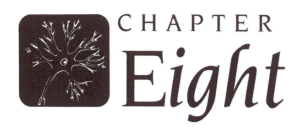

C H A P T E R

Eight

Assessment Strategies: A Sense of Perspective

The terms dysarthria and apraxia invoke a sense of difficulty when considering assessment strategies. This difficulty is more apparent than real. The assessment of the child with a developmental motor speech disorder is no more difficult than the assessment of any other child with a communication problem, and in some instances, it is much easier. After a few moments of observation and interactive communication with the child, many communicative strengths and weaknesses become obvious. The presence of multiple articulation errors, dysprosody, motoric struggle during speech, limited grammatical form, and spared comprehension of spoken language are common observations. Following this initial period of observation, various assessment protocols are used to document, with some objectivity it is hoped, both the strengths and weaknesses of the communicative profile. What seems to be missing in the clinical approach to assessment of developmental motor speech disorders is a sense of perspective: "What do I evaluate and where do I begin?" Certain aspects of developmental motor speech disorders merit close inspection: motor and motor speech functions, articulation/phonological performance, language performance, and potential interactions among these aspects of communication. At times, additional deficits will require clinical focus such as poor attention, memory limitations, psychosocial characteristics, and others. However, these do not present any more difficulty in the assessment of the child with a developmental motor speech disorder than for any other communicatively impaired child. The fear and mystique surrounding the assessment of the child with a developmental motor speech disorder can be reduced by meeting the problem head on. This chapter presents five aspects of the evaluation for developmental motor speech disorders: clinical history and initial observations, motor performance, motor speech performance, articulation/phonologic performance, and language performance. The chapter concludes with suggestions for organizing evaluation sessions and decision-making strategies based on the motolinguistic model.

Clinical History and Initial Observations

Background Questionnaires

Much can be learned about any developmental communicative disorder even before the child is seen. Hospital consults, letters of referral, and parent or teacher concerns all are useful sources of information. Wherever and whenever possible, a background questionnaire completed by the child's parents prior to the clinical examination will serve as a useful information resource. A sample questionnaire is included as Appendix A. Although brief, such surveys help to paint a picture of the child and his or her communicative environment. Answers to the questions on this form provide information about the basic concerns of the parent and/or child, including potential reactions by the child to the communicative deficits. Basic developmental milestones are reviewed including babbling and use of gestures to communicate. Family characteristics and, for older children, academic performance also are reviewed. Questions should be included on feeding and swallowing history to address the possibility of a dysarthria or a dysphagia component in children with a potential apraxia of speech. The overall purpose of this information is to paint a larger picture of the communicative difficulties and their ramifications for the child's day-to-day functioning prior to the clinical assessment. This strategy often helps to streamline the clinical evaluation. Sometimes limited information is available and/or it is not possible to obtain a completed background questionnaire from the family. In these cases, other sources of information may prove useful. Referral letters from pediatricians or pediatric neurologists often contain little specific information on speech-language, but do review the child's medical status and developmental milestones as well as providing an opinion regarding the nature of communication difficulties. Referrals from psychologists often document intelligence and psychoeducational considerations that have direct bearing on communicative difficulties. Information also is available for the child who is identified on the basis of speech-language screening programs. Each of these sources of information is valuable in developing initial clinical hypotheses and formulating a plan for the clinical evaluation.

Initial Observations

All clinicians are pressed for time, some more than others, but it is strongly advised that a few minutes be set aside to observe the child in a low-structured (informal) communicative situation. These few minutes may be invaluable in adjusting clinical hypotheses based on preconceived notions and/or in adjusting impressions formed about the child from prior information. Certainly, these few minutes will be useful in designing the remainder of the evaluation. Specific observations may pertain directly to the child with a developmental motor speech disorder. Although not an exhaustive list, some suggestions for informal observation are offered in Table 8–1.

The basic components of the evaluation process are included in this observation checklist. These observations begin at first sighting or hearing of the child. An occupational therapist who worked extensively with children with motor disorders once commented that she could pick out an apraxic child at first sight (here referring to a generalized apraxia). "The shirt is buttoned in-

Table 8–1. Suggestions for pre-evaluation clinical observations of children with developmental motor speech disorders.

Nonspeech Motor Functions	*Articulation/Phonological Performance*
General Sensorimotor Organization	Amount of Verbal Output
Posture and gait	Quiet, reluctant to speak
Movement patterns	Highly interactive
Gross and fine sensorimotor	Overall intelligibility
coordination	Type of Errors
Oral Sensorimotor Organization	Indication of "dominant" error type
Overt paresis—asymmetry in the	
mechanism	*Language Performance*
Mouth posture	Comprehension
Drooling, mastication, swallow-	Understand basic questions,
ing, etc.	instructions
	Answers, interacts appropriately
Speech Motor Functions	Expression
Nonspeech Indicators	Gestures and/or verbal output
Struggle, strain during speech	Type of utterances (single words,
Visible groping of the oral	sentences, etc.)
articulators	
Speech Indicators	*Other Observations*
Fluency of speech	Attention
Prosodic deviations	Focus, shift, sustain
Hyper-Hyponasality	Easily distracted/self-distracted
Voice deviations	Reaction to Speech
	Shy, withdrawn, crying
	Aggressive
	Other

correctly, the zipper is down, the shoes are untied or unevenly fastened with velcro, the glasses are on crooked and the child has a generally disorganized look." Unfortunately (perhaps fortunately for the child), children with a focal developmental motor speech disorder typically do not demonstrate this degree of overt motor disarray. However, certain general aspects of motor function should be considered in addition to basic communicative interaction and style. Posture and gait should be noted. Mouth posture (open, closed) and the presence of facial paresis and drooling should be noted. During speech attempts is there any suggestion of struggle, groping activity within the oral speech mechanism, dysprosody, nasality, or voice deviations? How verbal is the child? Is he or she reticent to speak, using only a few single words, or is communication approached with reckless abandon? Are gestures used instead of words? What type of articulation errors seem the most prominent? Does the child understand basic questions and attempt to answer? Are attention mechanisms strong or limited? Does the child focus, sustain, and shift attention appropriately? Finally, what, if any, is the child's reaction to attempts to encourage speech? Experience has revealed a wide range of reactions on the part of children with developmental motor speech disorders. These range from putting the head on the table to crying to an extreme case in which the child vomited during each session when asked to perform speech tasks presumably beyond his ability level. Each clinician will form his or her own list of important mental observations, and different observations will be made from each encounter with these children. However, the use of a brief, interactive observation is recommended to confirm prior impressions and to facilitate structuring the remaining evaluation.

Structuring the Evaluation

Conceiving of the evaluation session (or sessions) as a connected and interactive series of mini-evaluations may be a useful strategy. As stated above, the five aspects to be evaluated include motor, motor speech, articulation/phonology, language, and "other." Table 8–2 presents suggested elements of each aspect of the basic evaluation.

One other consideration should be addressed before jumping into the evaluation proper. The sequence of events should be determined with consideration for the child's perceived abilities including interaction and cooperation for various communicative tasks. Also, it should be determined whether the evaluation can realistically be completed in one session or will require multiple sessions to ensure the child's cooperation? No set answers exists to these issues because clinical environments vary as do children's abilities. Many times it is advisable to begin the evaluation with tasks that do not require speech or complex motor responses from the child. In other situations, it may be necessary to complete the speech assessment initially followed by the non-

Table 8-2. Basic components of the evaluation of developmental motor speech disorders.

Motor	Articulation/Phonological Assessment
Oral Structural-Functional Examination	Standardized Articulation Tests
Anatomy and asymmetry	Objective severity assessment
Basic movement characteristics	Normative comparison
(range, speed, etc.)	Typically sound based
Reflexes	Phonological Analysis
Lingual/labial-mandibular	Patterns of errors
dependency	Choice of elicitation technique
Volitional Oral Movements (Praxis)	Performance Load Effects
Traditional praxis examination	Performance at increasing levels
Volitional oral movement task	of complexity
(single—sequential)	Other Phonological Functions
Volitional Limb Movements (Praxis)	Parallels with written language
Test of limb apraxia	deficits
Fist-Edge-Palm task	Internal phonological processing
Communicative gestures	
	Language Assessment
Motor Speech	Comprehension
Basic Performance Patterns	Semantic, syntactic comprehension
Prosody, fluency	Effect of increased length of input
Nasality, voice deviations	Expression
Maximum performance tests	Standardized tests
Speech Diadochokinesis	Interactive conversation and/or
Alternate motion rate	extended description
Sequential motion rate	Bottom up interference
Bite block effects	
	Extended Evaluations
	Attention, perceptual, memory
	functions, etc.
	Intelligence, educational evaluation
	Medical evaluation
	Extended sensorimotor evaluation

speech tasks. A strategy for younger and/or communicatively frustrated children developed through experience is to begin with a relatively simple nonspeech pointing task such as a receptive vocabulary protocol, especially if the child is tentative about the examination process. This might be followed by an intermingling of speech and nonspeech tasks to avoid putting the child into a set of tasks with a high probability for failure. The ultimate goal is to create a situation in which the child is cooperating fully with each task presented. Even with manipulation of the task schedule, it may be necessary to provide ample breaks between tasks or even to schedule multiple sessions to complete the entire evaluation.

Evaluation of Nonspeech Motor Functions

If initial observations indicate a generalized apraxia or suggestion of paresis outside of the speech mechanism, referral to a qualified occupational and/or physical therapist or physician might be indicated. If the clinical situation permits, speech-language pathologists might evaluate gross and fine motor skills themselves. The focus of this section is on nonspeech oral motor and limb functions that may relate to the various motor speech disorders or have importance for treatment planning and implementation.

Structural-Functional Examination of the Speech Mechanism

Basic Observations and Reflex Testing

It is inappropriate to assume, even in the presence of strong observational evidence or prior report, that the oral speech mechanisms are adequate. As indicated repeatedly in earlier chapters, the presence of a developmental motor speech disorder does not preclude the possibility of an accompanying structural deficit in the peripheral mechanism. In most instances, examination of oral structures requires only a few minutes. A good rule of thumb is to look for evidence of asymmetry in paired, symmetrical structures. This cursory examination is important not only for identifying accompanying deficits, but also for confirming or excluding the presence of paresis in orofacial muscles used for speech production. The presence of paresis would be indicative of direct motor pathology potentially associated with dysarthria. Abnormal reflexes in the orofacial region also may be identified in dysarthric (and some apraxic) children. In cases of congenital suprabulbar paresis, abnormal reflexes would be associated with upper motor neuron (UMN) deficits. Worster-Drought (1974) emphasizes the jaw jerk and snout reflexes as potentially abnormal findings in congenital suprabulbar paresis. The jaw jerk is elicited by asking the patient to relax the mandible with examiner support. The examiner then taps the mental process downward. An exaggerated closure or bite would be an indication of a hyperactive jaw jerk response. Obviously, this procedure would be difficult to complete on most, especially younger, children. The snout response also is sometimes associated with UMN dysfunction. This reflex is elicited by tapping on the upper or lower lip. The abnormal response is marked by contraction of both the upper and lower lips as well as muscles at the base of nose. This gives the appearance of a "snout." In some cases the gag reflex may be reduced, absent, or even exaggerated. The gag reflex is elicited by mechanical stimulation (usually a tongue blade) to the base of the tongue near the valleculae. Remember that a reduced, absent, or exaggerated gag reflex in the absence of other neurological signs may indicate nothing. An asymmetrical gag reflex typically indicates lower motor neuron or sensory deficits. Additional signs of abnormal vegetative functions in the orofacial mechanisms may be observed during a short feeding evaluation. Signs of poor oral control of food or liquid or abnormal mastication and/or swallowing functions may be indicative of motor deficits likely to be associated with dysarthria or possibly some forms of apraxia of speech.

Strength, Range of Movement and Speed

A variety of tasks may be attempted to identify deviations in strength, range of movement, and/or speed of movement among the oral speech mechanisms. These are common techniques found in most structural-functional protocols examining the oral mechanisms. One modification that may be useful is to use a bite block to stabilize the mandible when evaluating lingual movements. This technique, recommended by Dworkin and Culatta (1980), may be useful in identifying structural or functional limitations in tongue movement. By stabilizing the mandible (see Chapter 5) limitations in volitional tongue movement may be more easily observed.

Hypernasality

Especially in instances where hypernasality is perceived, a detailed functional examination of the velopharyngeal port is indicated. In some cases this examination may go beyond the confines of a perceptually based speech examination of velopharyngeal functions. In these cases, aerodynamic, videofiberoptic, and/or fluorographic examinations may be required to determine whether increased nasality is the result of structural or functional deficits or both.

Voice

A cursory voice examination also should be completed. This examination should include observation of basic voice characteristics as well as maximum phonation time and the ability to manipulate pitch and loudness characteristics. Clinicians should note any obvious changes in voice characteristics associated with syllable or word attempts (including conversation) versus isolated vowel productions.

Interpretations

Most of the time, the results of the structural-functional examination of the speech mechanisms will alert clinicians to the possibility of a dysarthria or a dysarthric component associated with a developmental apraxia of speech. Many children with a developmental apraxia of speech will reveal few, if any, limitations on this portion of the clinical evaluation. Perhaps the most frequently encountered deficits include limited independent lingual motion and changes in nasality and/or voice characteristics, especially when the speech mechanism is stressed.

Volitional Oral Movements

Preliminary Concerns

Beyond the basics of "stick out your tongue and pucker your lips," clinicians must evaluate some aspects of praxis or volitional movement control. Traditional tests of volitional oral movements often involve meaningful or representative movements such as "show me how you kiss a baby" or "show me how you lick an ice cream cone" in addition to nonrepresentational movements such as "stick out your tongue" (De Renzi, Pieczuro, & Vignolo, 1966; Spriestersbach, Morris, & Darley, 1978). Some protocols require the production of sequences of these movements (LaPointe & Wertz, 1974; Yoss & Darley, 1974a). Most of these protocols are presented as an auditory command or as an examiner-provided example (essentially an imitation task). Some investigators (e.g., Yoss & Darley, 1974a) have used a combination of verbal command and/or demonstration in testing volitional oral movement control. In Chapters 3 and 5, the procedure used by Mateer (Mateer & Kimura, 1977; Mateer, 1978) was described. This procedure is attractive as a clinical protocol to evaluate volitional oral movement control in children. It incorporates nonrepresentational movements, limiting the potential for the child's semantic interpretation of the movement to influence performance (Cermak, 1985). It is a relatively short procedure that is not likely to induce fatigue as a confounding variable. And, perhaps most importantly, it systematically evaluates single and sequential movement performances. In this regard, the procedure may be used as a traditional evaluation of oral apraxia, to evaluate the influence of sequential complexity on performance of the same oral movements, and to evaluate potential sequencing or performance load influences during sequencing of different movements.

Stimulus Presentation and Reliability of Scoring

Crary and his colleagues (Crary & Anderson, 1990; Crary & Towne, 1984) have used this procedure to evaluate volitional oral movement performance in children with developmental motor speech disorders (see Chapter 5). Prior to clinical application, manner of stimulus presentation and reliability of scoring were evaluated. To evaluate potential influences from different methods of stimulus presentation, the procedure was administered to 12 children (6 apraxic and 6 normal) under three conditions: direct imitation of the examiner, picture demonstration (child is shown a picture of posture[s] and asked to perform the same movement), and from memory following picture stimuli. The results of this pilot study are presented in Figure 8–1. Although each condition elicited more errors from the children with an apraxia of speech, the picture stimuli condition best differentiated normal from disordered speakers. The picture stimuli condition also affords the highest degree of examiner control. Less variability is expected among administrations of this task using picture stimuli compared to examiner modeling. It was also the only condition in which the children with normal speech-language abilities did not demonstrate a high error percentage on one or more of the complexity levels. For these reasons, the picture stimuli condition was used in the studies described in Chapter 5 and is recommended for clinical evaluation of volitional oral movement performance.

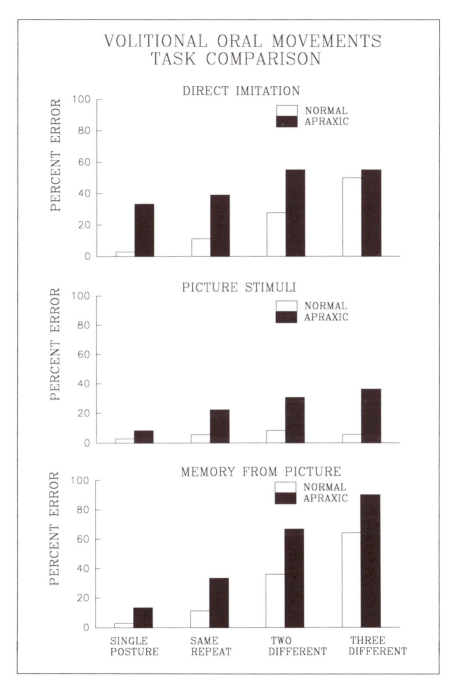

Figure 8–1. Performance of 12 children (6 with apraxia of speech and 6 with normal speech-language performance) on the volitional oral movement task under three conditions: direct imitation of examiner model, picture stimuli, and memory from picture stimuli.

Reliability of scoring also was addressed in pilot research. Two separate data sets were analyzed for scoring reliability. Data from 10 subjects from the procedural pilot study (above) were re-evaluated by two independent judges. Using a three-way comparison (original judge and two independent judges), average agreement on judgement of correct or incorrect responses among the 10 children was 92% with a range from 75% to 100% agreement. The second reliability analysis was presented in the Crary and Anderson (1990) study. Two independent judges scored responses from 20 children (10 apraxic and 10 normal) from videotaped administration of the picture stimuli version of this task. Comparison of correct/incorrect responses yielded an average of 92.5% agreement. (This figure includes results of hand movement task—see below.) Because this study also evaluated type of error in a movement task, judges' agreement was calculated for error type analysis. For 12 error types the average agreement was 85% (including the hand movement task). These data suggest that clinicians should be able to reliably judge responses on the oral movement task (and the hand movement task) as correct or incorrect. Furthermore, if error analysis is completed, moderate reliability may be expected.

Procedures

The administration of the volitional oral movement task is quite simple. Each child is shown a series of 24 photographs each depicting either a single facial posture (six photographs) or a sequence of facial postures (six photographs for each of three complexity levels: same posture repeated three times, two different postures, and three different postures). The facial postures include: protrude the lips (pucker), lateralize the tongue outside the mouth, elevate the tongue outside the mouth, open the mouth, protrude the tongue, and bite the lower lip. The photographs used in the Crary studies were 8½ X 11 black and white pictures provided by Catherine Mateer. Prior to task administration, each child is given instructions to make the face or faces presented in each picture. Crary and Anderson (1990) developed a set of training pictures of an adult female closing one eye, both eyes, or keeping both eyes open to demonstrate the expected responses at each level of sequential complexity. Each photograph is presented individually. Videotaping the child's responses is recommended whenever possible to minimize scoring mistakes. The order of presentation proceeds from single postures to the same posture repeated three times to two different postures to three different postures. The sheet presented in Figure 8–2 is used to score responses.

To interpret performance of this task based on the motolinguistic model, it is useful to note the presence of sequencing errors versus other error types. This is easily accomplished by writing the initials of each target movement on the lines provided on the score sheet along with notation regarding observed error types. Error type notations may be placed in a location depicting their occurrence in the response. For example, if groping is noted between the first and second postures, a "G" may be written in the space between the first and

```
NAME:

DATE:

                    EVALUATION OF ORAL MOVEMENTS (PRAXIS)

                              Single Movements

Movement                           +/-                    (Comments)

Protrude Lips (PL)               _____
Protrude Tongue (PT)             _____
Open Mouth (OM)                  _____
Lateralize Tongue (LT)           _____
Elevate Tongue (ET)              _____
Bite Lower Lip (BL)              _____


                    Three Movement Sequence (Same Movement)

Sequence                        Response                   Score

PL    PL    PL            _____   _____   _____         _____
OM    OM    OM            _____   _____   _____         _____
PT    PT    PT            _____   _____   _____         _____
BL    BL    BL            _____   _____   _____         _____
ET    ET    ET            _____   _____   _____         _____
LT    LT    LT            _____   _____   _____         _____


                    Two Movement Sequence (Different Movements)

Sequence                        Response                   Score

PL    ET                 _____   _____                 _____
OM    LT                 _____   _____                 _____
LT    BL                 _____   _____                 _____
ET    PL                 _____   _____                 _____
LT    OM                 _____   _____                 _____
BL    LT                 _____   _____                 _____


                    Three Movement Sequence (Different Movements)

Sequence                        Response                   Score

PT    OM    BL           _____   _____   _____         _____
PL    OM    LT           _____   _____   _____         _____
PT    PL    BL           _____   _____   _____         _____
BL    OM    PT           _____   _____   _____         _____
LT    OM    PL           _____   _____   _____         _____
BL    PL    PT           _____   _____   _____         _____
```

Figure 8–2. Sample of score sheet used to score the volitional oral movement task.

second response columns. A single "+" or "−" score is used to provide a quick tally of overall performance (number or percent correct). If the child self-corrects an incorrect movement, a correct response is scored. Incorrect responses may come in many forms. Following scoring from De Renzi, et al. (1966) and Roy and Square (1985), Crary and Anderson (1990) used 12 error categories to score incorrect responses. These are listed in Table 8–3. Figure 8–3 displays a completed score form. The child depicted in this profile would be considered to demonstrate a planning variant of apraxia with the presence of mild sequencing difficulties in addition to signs of oral apraxia (primarily groping). In this instance, groping was not considered an error if the resulting posture was correct.

Table 8–3. Definition of error types used to score the volitional oral and hand movement tasks.

Error Type	Definition
All Levels	
Groping (G)	Searching movements with the tongue, lips, fingers, or hand.
Incorrect Posture (IP)	Production of a posture other than the target posture.
Perseveration (P)	Production of an immediately preceding target posture.
Partial Response (PR)	Incomplete production of a posture.
Exaggerated Response (ER)	Over emphasized response.
Slow Initiation (SI)	Hesitation prior to initiation of response.
Slow Release (SR)	Prolonged posture. Delay in releasing a posture.
Vocalization (V)	Verbal description of a posture rather than face or hand production of posture.
Use of Hand (H)	Use of hand(s) to assist in facial postures or uninvolved hand to assist in hand task.
Sequential Tasks Only	
Slow Transition (ST)	Delay between production of successive postures in a sequence.
Addition of Unrelated Posture (UP)	Production of an extra posture not in the target sequence.
Sequence Error (S)	Production of the target sequence in the wrong order.

Source: Adapted from Crary and Anderson (1990).

Hand Movement Task

Preliminary Concerns

As depicted in Chapter 5, evaluation of volitional limb (hand) movements may be useful in interpreting a child's motor performance in reference to the motolinguistic model. However, there is also a more generic clinical reason for evaluating volitional limb movement control in some children with a developmental motor speech disorder. There are cases of severe speech production deficits in which alternate forms of communication involving limb movements may be considered. In these situations, examination of volitional limb movement performance will be a mandatory part of the clinical examination. A variety of volitional hand movement or limb praxis tasks may be used. In consideration of the motolinguistic model, Crary and Towne (1984) and

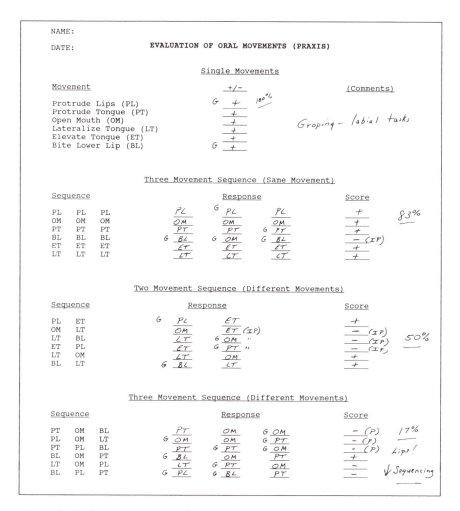

Figure 8–3. Sample of a completed score sheet for the volitional oral movement task.

Crary and Anderson (1990) used a modification of Luria's (1980) fist-edge-palm task. As the name implies, this task incorporates three hand positions, fist, edge, and palm, alone and in combination. This task is similar to the oral movement task in that children are asked to produce isolated and sequential hand postures. The task is somewhat different in that the children are able to watch their hands during this task, but they are not able to watch their faces during the oral movement task. This procedural difference may contribute to some of the apparent discrepancies among motor tasks discussed in Chapter 5. Despite these differences, the hand movement task is organized similarly to the oral movement task, permitting evaluation of both single and sequential hand movements.

One additional aspect should be considered in the evaluation of hand/limb movement performance. Specifically, in instances in which some form of gestural communication is being considered as a therapy technique or as a functional mode of communication, it would seem important to evaluate the child's performance on more complex, semantically potent movements. Just as semantic interpretation is kept at a nil or minimum level when attempting to evaluate motor performance, it is important to evaluate the influence of semantic interpretation as well as motor performance when considering use of gestural modes of communication.

Procedural Considerations and Scoring Reliability

Preliminary studies on this procedure evaluated differences attributed to hand use and scoring reliability. A comparison of performances with the right versus left hand in six apraxic and six normal children revealed only minimal differences in the mean number of errors produced by either group between the two hands. There was no consistent pattern of superior or inferior performance from one hand versus the other. Reliability for correct and incorrect responses and error type classification in the Crary and Anderson (1990) study was included with results of the oral movements task (see above). A separate reliability computed from the scores of three independent judges on performance of 10 children (5 apraxic and 5 normal) indicated 99% percent agreement on correct/incorrect judgments. This finding may suggest that the hand movement task is slightly easier to score than the oral movement task. One reason for this may be that both apraxic and normal children make fewer errors on this procedure than on the oral movement task (Crary & Anderson, 1990; Crary and Towne, 1984).

Procedures

The hand movement task is organized identically to the oral movement task with the exception that, because there are only three basic hand postures, there is a total of 18 stimuli versus 24. A score sheet is used to tally responses, and videotaping is recommended whenever possible to facilitate accurate scoring. Similar to the oral movements task, primary concern focuses on deficits at the single posture level, repetitions of the same posture, and sequencing of two and three different postures. The same scoring conventions and error categories used in the oral movement task are used to score the hand movement task. Figure 8–4 presents a score form for the hand movement task.

Some Cautionary Advice

The protocols for evaluation of volitional oral and hand movements presented here (and for that matter any task of volitional movement that has not been rigorously studied) should be applied clinically only with a healthy sense of their limitations. Aside from the limited studies on adults and children dis-

```
NAME:

DATE:

                    EVALUATION OF HAND MOVEMENTS (PRAXIS)

                              Single Movements

    Movement                        +/-                    (Comments)

    Side (S)                        ____
    Palm (P)                        ____
    Fist (F)                        ____


                    Three Movement Sequence (Same Movement)

    Sequence                      Response                    Score

    SSS            ____    ____    ____                       ____
    PPP            ____    ____    ____                       ____
    FFF            ____    ____    ____                       ____


                Two Movements Sequence (Different Movements)

    Sequence                      Response                    Score

    SP             ____    ____                               ____
    FP             ____    ____                               ____
    SF             ____    ____                               ____
    PS             ____    ____                               ____
    PF             ____    ____                               ____
    FS             ____    ____                               ____


                Three Movement Sequence (Different Movements)

    Sequence                      Response                    Score

    SPF            ____    ____    ____                       ____
    PSF            ____    ____    ____                       ____
    FPS            ____    ____    ____                       ____
    PFS            ____    ____    ____                       ____
    SFP            ____    ____    ____                       ____
    FSP            ____    ____    ____                       ____
```

Figure 8–4. Sample of score sheet used to score the volitional hand movement task.

cussed in Chapters 3 and 5, few, if any studies have evaluated the properties of these procedures. They are not standardized motor assessment protocols. No published study has evaluated the performance of speech-language and motor normal children at different ages. The majority of the children in the Crary studies were between the ages of 4 and 8 years, with an average age between 4½ and 5½. Until more extensive research is completed on the potential of these procedures to measure various aspects of volitional oral and hand motor performances, it is strongly recommended that they be considered descriptive assessment tools. To attempt to use these protocols to distinguish normal from abnormal motor performance would be inappropriate.

However, these protocols may be useful in describing patterns of volitional oral and hand movements, especially in situations where systematic evaluation of both single and sequential movement patterns is considered important.

Evaluation of Motor Speech Functions

Initial Observations and Decisions

During initial observation and interaction with the child, impressions will be formed concerning motor speech deficits. Obvious struggle or groping of oral articulators during speech may suggest an apraxic component. Obvious paresis or limited range and/or speed of movement during speech may suggest a dysarthric component. All or any of these symptoms may contribute to a dysprosody as well as deficient speech articulation. Abnormal voice production should be noted as well as deviations in nasality. Simply observing the deficits is insufficient. The clinician must attempt to determine the performance capabilities of the various components of speech mechanism. Kent, Kent, and Rosenbek (1987) claim that "maximum performance tests find some of their most frequent clinical applications in screening and in the assessment of motor speech disorders" (p. 381). Similar to the procedures described for the assessment of volitional motor function, tests of maximum performance of speech also are limited by a relative paucity of standardized procedures. However, these procedures often have the benefit of multiple studies evaluating both normal and abnormal performances. In this regard, tests of maximum performance for speech functions seem to be one scientific step ahead of the tests of volitional motor performance described in this chapter.

Some tests of motor speech performance, maximum or otherwise, are not realistically completed in a variety of clinical environments, primarily due to the need for expensive equipment to complete these procedures. However, most clinicians, regardless of environment, are able to evaluate many aspects of maximum speech performance including: maximum phonation duration, maximum fricative duration and s/z ratio, pitch and loudness control (at least a subjective perceptual judgment) and diadochokinetic performance. Kent, Kent, and Rosenbek (1987) offer a thorough review of these and other maximum performance tasks. Given the predominance of speech diadochokinetic performances among studies of children with developmental motor speech disorders and the potential contribution of these procedures toward motolinguistic profiling, procedures and interpretation of speech diadochokinetic testing are offered.

Speech Diadochokinetic Testing

Procedural Decisions

Speech diadochokinesis assessments are a standard technique in most speech evaluation batteries. Kent, Kent, and Rosenbek (1987) refer to these proce-

dures as "Maximum Repetition Rate" (MRR). Individuals are asked to repeat either single syllables (alternate motion rate) or syllable sequences
(sequential motion rate). Consider two basic questions when selecting tasks
of speech diadochokinesis: Which syllables will be used and how will the responses be scored? The answer to the first question depends on the goals of
the examiner and the abilities of the child. Typically, the syllables "puh",
"tuh," and "kuh" alone and in two- and three-syllable sequences are used to
evaluate MRR. However, many clinicians, finding these syllables difficult or
impossible for a child to produce, will use words such as "pattycake" or "but-
tercup." Also, children unable to produce the voiceless consonants in this
task may replace them with voiced cognates (b, d, g). Clinicians may inten-
tionally vary the target stimuli to examine diadochokinetic performance
from the perspective of various speech "valves." For example, "huh" may be
used to study laryngeal performance, "fuh" may be used to study labiodental
placement, and so on. These applications are rare, however, and typically employed only with a specific question in mind.

Scoring Decisions

Acceptable Responses. The scoring issue overlaps with the choice of
target syllables. There are two basic scoring issues. First, what is an acceptable
response for this task? If the target is a voiceless consonant paired with a vowel (puh) and the response is a voiced consonant paired with a vowel (buh), it
is unacceptable to apply any available norms for "puh" to the voiced responses.
This does not mean that the response pattern is uninformative. Such deviations are often very informative. However, clinicians must keep in mind that
10 repetitions of "pattycake" do not equal 10 repetitions of "puh-tuh-kuh."
At least, there is no research that suggests the two responses are equivalent.
Another question of acceptable response is the issue of interruptions created by a breath. Kent and colleagues (1987) caution clinicians to take care
"that the number of syllables does not exceed the subject's capability on a
single breath . . ." (p. 379). However, the published procedure by Fletcher
(1972) contains no such warning among its instructions. Clinicians certainly
should make note of variations in performance secondary to breathing (as well
as other factors such as articulatory groping) when scoring these procedures.

Count-By-Time or Time-By-Count. Two methods may be used for
scoring diadochokinetic speech rates: count-by-time and time-by-count. In
the first method, count the number of syllables produced in a given time
frame. These results might be expressed as the total number of syllables produced within that time (10 puh-tuh-kuhs in 10 seconds) or as syllables per
second (1.0 puh-tuh-kuh/second). This procedure is slightly cumbersome
because clinicians must count syllables and watch a stop watch at the same
time and then compute the ratio. Conversely, this procedure may be useful
in cases of severe speech disorder, especially if a child is unable to produce
the required number of syllables for the other scoring procedure. In those instances, the count-by-time ratio accompanied by the total number of sylla-

bles produced may serve as an indication of MRR. The other scoring procedure, time-by-count, was made clinically popular by Fletcher (1972). In this procedure, a required number of syllables is produced, and the resultant time in seconds is measured. For example, 20 repetitions of "puh" in 5 seconds. This procedure is somewhat less cumbersome than the count-by-time procedure, and its popularity may be attributed partially to a convenient single scoring sheet containing normative performance data from children ages 6 through 13. Unfortunately, there are few, if any, normative performance data for children below 5 or 6 years of age. Given the variability seen among normal speakers (see Kent, Kent, & Rosenbek, 1987) on this task and the expected increase in variability among younger children, clinicians should exercise caution when interpreting performance of younger children.

Beyond the Basics: Error Patterns and Bite Blocks

Error Patterns

Beyond comparison of the individual child's performance on speech diadochokinetic tasks to normative data, other descriptive analyses may prove useful in cases of developmental motor speech disorders. In Chapter 5 two issues were considered: pattern of performance and potential influence of mandibular stabilization via a bite block. The pattern of individual performance may implicate deficient underlying speech processes and assist in profiling the child along the lines suggested by the motolinguistic model. For example, a child who produces slow alternate motion rates and is unable to produce any or produces a limited number of sequential targets, may demonstrate an executive apraxic variant. The dysarthric child may produce a slow, regular cadence across both alternate and sequential motion tasks. Conversely, toward the planning end of the continuum, clinicians might expect to see intact alternate motion tasks with impaired performance on sequential tasks.

Bite Blocks

Bite blocks also may be useful in evaluating diadochokinetic performance in children with developmental motor speech disorders. Recall from Chapter 5 that certain adults with apraxia of speech demonstrated relatively normal diadochokinetic performances when a bite block was not used, but demonstrated impaired performance not characteristic of normal speakers when a bite block was used to stabilize the mandible. Children with apraxia of speech also demonstrated a deterioration in diadochokinetic performance when a bite block was used to stabilize the mandible during the speech tasks. Bite blocks may be fashioned individually from hard plastic or hard rubber. Netsell (1985) describes a technique to construct bite blocks out of dental impression compound. A tongue blade is notched for contact with the incisors as an initial gauge of jaw opening. Netsell recommends an interincisal distance of 8–10 mm for adults and 5–8 mm for children 3- to 10-years-old. This is based on clinical impressions of one third of the patient's maximal interincisor distance. No hard and fast rule exists for determining the correct size of a bite block for a given individual. A block of soft dental compound is fashioned and placed posterior to the lower canine incisor. With the tongue blade in place, the person "bites" until maximum closure is obtained against the tongue blade. The block is then removed from the open mouth and the excess material is trimmed away. Strong string is attached to the block as a retrieval mechanism to prevent accidental choking. This technique provides an individual fit for bite blocks for each individual. If dental compound is not readily available, an acceptable substitute may be found in your local sporting goods store. Mouth protectors are firm plastic dental inserts that soften when placed in hot water. A piece of this device may be cut away, softened, secured with strong fishing line (emphasis on strong!), and fashioned into a bite block, much the same way as Netsell uses dental compound. If neither of these options is realistic, a piece of hard rubber may suffice.

Once fashioned, a bite block may be used to stabilize the mandible to evaluate speech and nonspeech motor functions. In addition to lingual-mandibular dependency, clinicians should evaluate lip-jaw dependencies. This is most easily noted during speech tasks requiring labial consonants (e.g., "Buy Bobby a poppy") (Netsell, 1985) or bilabial syllables in the diadochokinetic tasks. Presently, no normative data are available for comparison of speech performance with and without a bite block. Clinicians must use clinical experience and common sense guidelines to interpret the respective performances. For example, if performance deteriorates when the bite block is placed, it is possible that the child is using excessive mandibular support to accomplish that specific task. If, however, performance improves when the block is placed, then the block may be acting to reduce or eliminate interfering jaw movements.

Evaluation of Articulation/Phonological Performance

Chapter 6 presented various phonological perspectives on the child with a developmental motor speech disorder. In most cases, multiple articulation errors will be obvious. In some cases, verbal output will be severely limited but articulation errors will still be evident. In other cases, the child will demonstrate significant verbal output, but be virtually unintelligible. The clinical assessment of articulation/phonological errors in developmental motor speech disorders is little different from assessment of any other child demonstrating speech articulation errors. What is different in many cases is the sheer number and severity of the errors and the presence of other accompanying deficits. Three aspects of articulation assessment should be pursued: standardized articulation testing, phonological pattern evaluation, and performance load considerations. At times it may prove useful to evaluate additional phonological aspects related to written language performance and/or "internal phonological processing."

Standardized Articulation Testing: Sounds and Severity

In this context, standardized articulation testing refers to the administration of articulation tests that follow fixed protocols and are norm-referenced. Typically, traditional tests evaluate a variety of preselected sounds in different positions within single words. Picture elicitation tasks are common. A primary benefit of these tests, aside from relatively easy administration, is that they provide a global severity index. This may be in the form of a raw score compared to chronological age norms (*Templin-Darley Screening Tests of Articulation*, Templin & Darley, 1960) or calculated percentile scores (*Goldman-Fristoe Test of Articulation*, Goldman & Fristoe, 1986). In many cases this type of documentation is desirable or necessary. Without further interpretation or application of additional procedures, however, these procedures may be insufficient for many aspects of clinical decision making (Garn-Nunn & Martin, 1992). This scenario may be especially true in cases of developmental motor speech disorders when multiple and severe articulation errors might be expected. In these instances, a more descriptive phonological analysis may prove beneficial.

Phonological Analyses: Patterns In the Chaos

Phonological analyses in general are procedures that look for organization among speech errors through the application of phonological rules. These procedures may take the form of distinctive features, phonological rules, or most recently phonological processes. Since the late 1970s phonological process analysis has become the dominant technique under the rubric of phonological analyses. Published literature contains ample documentation of the clinical benefits of these procedures. In certain cases, however, it may be a more efficient clinical strategy to document what the child produces correctly rather than to generate an exhaustive list of errors. Consider the child who produces only voiced labial sounds and back vowels for all word attempts. Certainly a phonological process analysis would reveal a long list of phonological errors, but is such an extensive analysis clinically efficient or even useful in such cases?

Questions regarding the elicitation technique on which the phonological process analysis is based should be addressed. The information presented in Chapter 6 suggested that different results may be obtained from different sampling techniques even when the same analysis procedures are used. This situation may influence important clinical decisions. In the Crary articles on phonological performance in developmental apraxia of speech (see Chapter Six) a phrase imitation task was selected as the procedure of choice to accomplish phonological process analysis. As presented in Chapter 6, this procedure may have certain advantages over conversation or single word elicitation techniques.

A *Phrase Imitation Procedure for Phonological Analysis*

The phrase imitation procedure used in the Crary series on phonological analysis is detailed here. Based on evaluations of both apraxic and normal-speaking children 13 phonological processes were selected for this procedure. They are listed in Chapter 6. Appendix B contains a more detailed description of each phonological process including specific errors that are to be included within each category. Phonological processes were categorized into the "basic six" and the "additional seven" based on their frequency of occurrence in normal and disordered speech and upon their frequency of selection as treatment targets. Appendix C contains the 60 phrases used in the analysis. Each phrase (with four exceptions) is three words long with the target word in the phrase-final stressed position. Each phrase is meaningful, and within that context attempts were made to precede each target with a neutral vowel. There are a few exceptions. The target words initially were taken from the *Blache Sound Properties Test* (Blache, 1978). Blache's list of target words was taken from traditional articulation tests and portrayed to evaluate all American-English phonemes in all potential syllabic positions. Eleven target words containing prevocalic two-segment clusters were added to Blache's list. Redundant patterns were eliminated, and the result was a 60-phrase procedure. The child is asked to repeat the examiner's model of each phrase. It is not necessary for the entire phrase to be repeated but this is usually the case. The clinician transcribes the production of the target word on the score sheet (Appendix D) for later analysis. Each production is evaluated in reference to syllable structure change (usually omissions) and sound substitutions. The target sound that is erred is then placed under the appropriate phonological process column. Figure 8–5 presents an example of a completed page from a score form. Appendix E presents a completed analysis.

Figure 8–5. Sample of a completed page from the phonological process analysis using the 60-item phrase imitation task.

TARGET	RESPONSE	SYLLABLE SHAPE	ERRORS (-)->(-)	DFC	DIC	CR	WSD	GR	ST	GL	FR	BK	PVV	LAB	VOC	VOW. NEUT.	OTHER
1. hæmɚ	hæmʊ		ɚ→ʊ													ɚ	
2. kom	to:	-m	k→t	m							k						
3. nɑf	na:	-f	dɪ→a	f												aɪ	
4. pɛnɪ																	
5. rɪŋ	wɪŋ		r→w							r							
6. pɪg	pɪ	-g	g	g													
7. pepɚ	pepʊ		ɚ→ʊ													ɚ	
8. tʌb																	
9. kɔfɪ	tɔfɪ		k→t								k						
10. væn	bæn		v→b						v								
11. muvɪz	muvi	-z	z		z												
12. bædʒɚ	bædʊ		dʒ→d / ɚ→ʊ								dʒ					ɚ	
13. fʌdʒ	fʌd		dʒ→d								dʒ						
14. zu	du		z→d								z						
15. ʃɝt	tʊt		ʃ→t / ɝ→ʊ								ʃ—ʃ					ɝ	
16. kʌp	tʌʔ	-p	k→t	p							k						
17. kʊkɪ	tʊtɪ		k→t / k→t								k / k						

Once all errors have been analyzed, numerical calculations are completed to obtain the relative strength (RS) value of each phonological process. This numerical procedure is simple and assists the clinician not only in developing a phonological profile of each child but in determining therapy targets and documenting change as a result of treatment. The total occurrences of each phonological process are tallied on the last page of the score form. These values are divided by the potential occurrences of each process to obtain the RS value. The potential occurrences of each phonological process in the phrase imitation procedure are listed in Appendixes D and E. If desirable or necessary, each phonological process may be evaluated in reference to the specific sounds that are substituted or omitted. This practice is useful in designing therapy targets. For clinicians collecting and analyzing conversational samples, the same procedures may be applied with the exception that the potential occurrences of each process must be recalculated for each conversational sample.

Performance Load Considerations: Now You See It, Now You Don't

In many respects the articulation/phonological assessment strategies described in this chapter incorporate performance load considerations. Speech production is evaluated at two levels: single words using a standard articulation test and at the phrase level using the phrase imitation task. Recall from Chapter 6 that in children with an apraxia of speech the phrase procedure resulted in more errors than the single word or the conversation techniques (when word selection was controlled). Furthermore, Crary and Comeau (1982) reported that results from the phrase imitation technique correlated highly (average correlation across 13 phonological processes = .97) with results from conversational sample analyses obtained from 20 preschool children with normal speech-language abilities. Thus, this procedure is expected to produce the same or similar phonological results to conversational analyses and provide the clinician control over target items and reduced time commitment for phonological evaluation.

If there is a need for additional performance load evaluation, it is suggested that such comparisons be completed on a select subset of phonological errors. Specifically, once a target error has been selected for therapy, clinicians may want to evaluate production of that phonological target in different contexts. Also, if there is confusion over which error to address first, performance load evaluation in a treatment context may be an important factor to consider. Depending on the treatment chosen, this "stimulability" assessment might incorporate any of the following production contexts: isolated sound, consonant-vowel combinations, meaningful words of different syllabic lengths, and/or sentences of various grammatical forms. In many cases the presence of a concomitant deficit language performance will implicate target grammatical forms to be used in the assessment of phonological performance load factors.

Other Phonological Functions: Transmodal Phonology

Especially in older, school-age children, it may be important to evaluate phonological functions in written language performances. Recall from Chapter 2 that there is evidence of a clinically significant relationship between spoken and written aspects of phonological function. The child who demonstrates severe phonological dysfunction in speech should be considered at risk for deficits involving written aspects of phonology. Even in children who do not demonstrate an educationally limiting dyslexia, a brief analysis of reading and writing styles may be beneficial in attempting to understand internal phonological processing. One clue to deficient phonological processing may be an over reliance on semantic processes during reading. This pattern, referred to as deep dyslexia, implies that the phonological system is bypassed as visual input directly accesses a semantic analyzer (Colheart, 1980). The same pattern has been referred to as "sight vocabulary" by Snowling and Stackhouse (1983) in their studies of reading abilities in children with apraxia of speech. Children using this strategy are able to read words presumably without the benefit of phonological analysis. Typically, successful reading depends on visually familiar words such as logos for commercial products or orthographically regular and simple words. Words demanding phonological interpretation (phonologically irregular forms such as those words containing silent letters) are particularly difficulty for the individual with deep dyslexia. Reading errors tend to reveal semantic paralexias (semantically related errors) or, less frequently, visually related errors.

Another technique that may prove informative in evaluating internal phonological processing is rhyming (Feinberg, Rothi, & Heilman, 1986; Nebes, 1975). Marquardt and Sussman (1991) reported that four apraxic children between the ages of 5 and 7 years had difficulty with four aspects of rhyming function. The focus of their comparisons was phonologic strategies rather than strategies involving other linguistic functions. Crary (1991) presented the case of a 9-year-old girl who had a history of severe speech deficits as a preschooler and had been considered to demonstrate an apraxia of speech. She had received many years of speech therapy, and at the time Crary saw her she produced only mild articulatory deviations on specific sounds. Her reading style reflected a deep dyslexia. She was able to read many regular words and advertisements of commercial items. Conversely, she was completely unable to read any words requiring phonological analysis. A rhyming task was administered in which a target word was provided followed by three choices. One choice rhymed with the target, one foil was semantically related, and one was not related phonologically or semantically (e.g., "toe": go, foot, door). The girl consistently chose the semantically related foil. Thus her reading style and her rhyming performance indicated a reliance on semantic processing and implied a deficit in phonological processing.

These limited observations should serve to stimulate clinical curiosity. There is some suggestion that deviant phonological development, seen prominently among children with developmental motor speech disorders, may contribute to, or perhaps result from, deficient internal phonological processing. This deficit, in turn, may contribute to other language performance deficits, specifically written language deficits. Furthermore, there is some suggestion from adult cases who have impaired linguistic processing following brain damage that deficient internal phonological processing may selectively impair oral naming and/or other spoken language functions (Caramazza, Berndt, & Basili, 1983). If such deficits are seen in individual children, clinicians should consider internal phonological processing limitations as a contributing factor. Unfortunately, no proven or even generally accepted procedures are available for evaluating internal phonological processing. However, with increasing interest in identifying processes contributing to speech-language deficits, such research and/or clinical protocols no doubt will appear soon.

Evaluation of Language Performance

At this juncture there should be little doubt that most, if not all, children with a developmental motor speech disorder will demonstrate some degree of accompanying language deficit. In most cases there will be a receptive-expressive split favoring language comprehension abilities. In some cases there will be a more global language deficit, and in other cases, there will be only subtle language problems. In this respect, evaluation of language performance is an important component in the assessment of any developmental motor speech disorder.

There are a multitude of language performance tests available addressing different chronological ages, aspects of language function, or language-related processes. The choice of a given procedure or combination of procedures rests with the experience and comfort level of the clinician. Because clinical procedures are constructed in various ways and purport to measure a variety of functions, clinicians should be aware of the strengths and limitations of any protocol as they may apply to a particular clinical assessment. Individual tests will not be described here. Rather, and more focal to the discussion of developmental motor speech disorders, a brief review of the rationale for evaluating certain aspects of language performance will be presented.

Language Comprehension

At least three areas of comprehension should be addressed: semantic comprehension, syntactic comprehension, and the influence of increased length of input (performance load). Receptive vocabulary or other tests of lexical knowledge may be used to infer extent of semantic knowledge. In most cases in which nonverbal intelligence is normal, we would expect age-appropriate performance in this area. Syntactic comprehension may be assessed via any number of published language comprehension tools. A variety of grammatical structures should be assessed from the basic grammatical morphemes to complex sentence structures. Length of input information may be more difficult to assess because grammatical complexity is often a confounding factor. In selecting procedures to evaluate influence of input, consider procedures that control for such variables.

At times it may be necessary to evaluate other input variables often considered "perceptual." These may include auditory and/or visual memory, discrimination, synthesis, sequencing, or any number of "lower level" information processing tasks. There is little information concerning the relevance of these functions to developmental motor speech disorders; however, individual studies have raised questions regarding performance, primarily of apraxic children, in these areas. When there is relevant clinical concern over potential limitations in these areas or when choice of treatment modality or procedure may depend on these functions, they should be evaluated thoroughly.

Language Expression

Given the frequency and severity of expressive language deficits noted among children with developmental motor speech disorders, significant detail should be provided in evaluating this area. Standardized tests of language expression may be a good place to begin. These procedures typically sample a broad variety of expressive language functions including semantic formulation and syntactic construction and compare the results to age-referenced norms. In this regard, clinicians administering these protocols obtain norm-referenced documentation of the expressive language deficit and an initial profile of strengths and weaknesses in the realm of language expression. A second step in the evaluation of expressive language functions would be a more detailed analysis of those strengths and weaknesses. In designing a treatment program to include aspects of language expression, clinicians will want to know which grammatic structures are correctly versus incorrectly produced and obtain information on length of utterance as well as grammatical complexity and semantic appropriateness. If, as is often the case, the assessment tool being used cannot be analyzed sufficiently to provide a meaningful analysis, a conversational or other "spontaneous" language sample may be helpful. Dollaghan, Campbell, and Tomlin (1990) have described a short video narration procedure that provides a controlled language sample in just under 2 minutes. Because the content of the sample is controlled, clinicians may be able to extract a wealth of information from samples obtained in this manner. Using this procedure also enhances clinicians' ability to compare samples obtained at different points in therapy or in modified contexts (i.e., reporting details from memory). The video narration task is deceptively simple, however, and younger children or children with very severe deficits and/or limited output may not be able to participate effectively in this procedure.

Consideration for Extended Evaluations

From time to time clinicians will encounter a child with a particularly severe developmental disorder encompassing more than motor speech deficits. Other times, the specifics of the motor speech disorder may be so severe that additional evaluation is indicated. In these instances, referral to any number of other professionals and/or team evaluation is indicated. Psychologists, occupational therapists, physical therapists, and physicians or other professionals may be consulted depending on the nature and severity of the problem. Considered the following case:

Janie was an 11-year-old who had a long history of speech therapy with a label of developmental apraxia of speech. Initial evaluation raised the issue of congenital suprabulbar paresis due to the presence of drooling, immature mastication patterns, hypernasality, and subtle asymmetry in the perioral and lingual musculature. Her speech was barely intelligible and deteriorated as rate increased. Her intelligence was in the normal range, and she was in a class for children with learning disabilities. Initial impressions included the observation that she was distractible and seemed socially immature. Other than deficits in the oral musculature she demonstrated no overt neuromotor deficits.

Although Janie had received an educational evaluation, she had not been evaluated by a neurologist. Given the impression of congenital suprabulbar paresis along with perceived attention deficits and social immaturity, a referral to a "neurodevelopmental team" was made. The neurologist on the team concurred with the impression of congenital suprabulbar paresis. Furthermore, EEG results revealed the presence of left temporal lobe seizures for which medication was prescribed. The team psychologist did not feel that Janie demonstrated an attention-deficit disorder but did agree that she was distractible and offered good suggestions for management in this area. In this case, the extended evaluation, initiated at the request of the speech-language pathologist, expanded the range of appropriate treatment options for this child.

Not every child requires referral beyond the speech-language pathologist. There are times, however, when outside opinions are mandatory for the successful management of a developmental motor speech disorder. Just when to refer depends on the experience, qualifications, and resources of the clinician and the availability of other professions.

Beyond Data Collection: Organizing Your Thoughts

Once the basic areas of motor function, speech performance, and language performance have been evaluated, it is necessary to organize the information toward its intended purpose—designing a successful treatment program. Assuming that sufficient evidence has been obtained to support the existence of a developmental motor speech disorder, two general questions are to be addressed: (1) What "type" of motor speech disorder does this child present? and (2) What are the specifics of the motor, speech, and language deficits?

The first question is considered in reference to the motolinguistic model. Three general categories might be considered: dysarthria, executive apraxia, and planning apraxia. Clinical reality often presents a mixture of symptomatology. When "mixed" cases are encountered, they should be identified as such. Still, it may prove useful to identify such cases as *primarily* dysarthric, executive, or planning. The focus is to profile the abilities of the child in order to facilitate decisions regarding appropriate treatment. As will be discussed in the next chapter, treatment programs have characteristics that make them more appropriate for one type of problem versus another. Matching the characteristics of the child to the characteristics of the treatment program often results in improved clinical efficiency.

Identifying the specifics of motor, speech, and language deficits is the first step toward developing a treatment program. Usually, treatment goals will go hand-in-hand with identified deficit areas. If a child demonstrates lingual-mandibular dependency and diadochokinetic performance is negatively influenced by mandibular stabilization, consideration should be given to a motor speech component in the treatment program. Phonological targets are selected from the results of the phrase imitation task with appropriate consideration for normal developmental patterns. Expressive language targets are selected from test results and based on developmental data, but with significant consideration given to phonological performance and the influence of bottom-up interference.

The preceding suggestions imply that the overall goal of treatment will be to improve speech intelligibility and spoken language performance. This is not always the case. Some children demonstrate so little verbal output that alternative sources of communication are indicated either in replacement of spoken functions or to facilitate their emergence. Prior to identifying treatment techniques, it is necessary to specify the goals of intervention. This point introduces Chapter 9, Intervention Strategies.

Clinically Relevant Highlights

Evaluation of the child with a suspected developmental motor speech disorder is a multifocal process. Consideration must be afforded to motor, speech, and language performances and potential positive or negative interactions among these areas. A few simple reminders may help.

1. Take a few moments to observe the child in a low-structured communicative interaction.
2. Structure the evaluation session(s) not to focus on overt deficits, but rather to obtain maximum cooperation from the child.
3. Complete systematic evaluations of motor, motor speech, articulation/phonological, and language aspects of communicative performance.
4. Look for potential interactions among these functions.
5. Get help by referral or from team evaluations when necessary.
6. **Organize evaluation findings into a framework that will facilitate the development of successful intervention strategies. The motolinguistic model is offered as an example of such a framework.**

Experienced clinicians will recognize the benefit of placing a perspective on the evaluation process. No single protocol will suffice to address all of the clinically relevant issues surrounding the evaluation of developmental motor speech disorders. Even with a loaded armamentarium of clinical perspective and protocols, there will be children who will tax even the best clinicians. Some days the dragon wins. Only through determined and systematic evaluation of these problems will successful intervention strategies emerge.

CHAPTER
Nine

Intervention Strategies: Making Changes That Matter

A Philosophy of Treatment

Faced with a child who demonstrates a probable developmental motor speech disorder, many clinicians (and parents) will ask: "How do I treat developmental apraxia of speech?" Unfortunately, there are many problems with this question. The preceding chapters in this text have repeatedly emphasized that there are many potential variants of developmental motor speech disorders. All too often the distinctions among variants are ignored, and a unitary approach to therapy is sought under the rubric of developmental apraxia of speech. A more appropriate clinical approach might be to consider what constitutes the apparent developmental motor speech disorder and to select and/or design an intervention strategy that matches the strengths and deficits profile of the child. In other words, rather than selecting a therapy strategy or technique based on personal beliefs surrounding a perceived unitary motor speech disorder (apraxia of speech), matching a treatment strategy to a profile of abilities and disabilities may prove a superior clinical approach. This is the philosophy of treatment inherent in the motolinguistic model. Rather than emphasizing a label to describe a difficult problem, the model emphasizes performance profiles that imply underlying strategies/deficits and directs clinicians toward appropriate therapy strategies. A brief review of traditional treatment philosophies and strategies will serve as a contrast to the approach advocated by the motolinguistic model. Prior to undertaking this discussion it is imperative to emphasize that there is more state-of-the-art than state-of-the-science in treatment strategies for children presenting any form of developmental motor speech disorder. Opinion and philosophy abound, but precious little controlled data are available to support the application of any intervention approach over any other approach. Faced with this scenario, clinicians frequently confess to frustration and confusion in selecting an appropriate treatment approach for children with developmental motor speech disorders. Although the approach advocated in this text offers a consistent philosophy to assessment and treatment of various developmental motor speech disorders, there is still a paucity of evidence to support the efficacy of suggested treatment strategies. In this respect, there is often more art than science involved when selecting a treatment approach or technique for any child with a developmental motor disorder.

Historical and Traditional Approaches

A Common Theme

The common theme among most traditional therapy approaches to developmental motor speech disorders is their "bottom-up" focus. Initial emphasis is placed on nonspeech oral movements and/or single consonant or vowel production, and the clinician and child attempt to build a complex and functional speech production system from that therapeutic groundwork. This strategy may be the approach of choice for some problems, but the consistent commentary that apraxic children fare poorly in therapy and require extensive and extended intervention does not speak well for this approach without qualification. A review of four publications will serve as an adequate overview of this approach to therapy in developmental motor speech disorders with an emphasis on developmental apraxia of speech.

Rosenbek, Hansen, Baughman, and Lemme (1974)

Rosenbek and colleagues approached developmental apraxia of speech from a focused motor speech deficit point of view. Their recommendations for therapy are, not surprisingly, strongly oriented toward the motor speech, bottom-up philosophy of intervention. Table 9–1 summarizes seven principles and procedures recommended by this group.

Goals

The initial item on their list is a goal of treatment; one that the authors recognize as commonplace and relevant to a wide variety of communication deficits. Some children may have such significant limitations within the motor

Table 9-1. Seven principles and procedures of treatment for developmental apraxia of speech recommended by Rosenbek, Hansen, Baughman, and Lemme (1974).

1. Help the child acquire as near normal volitional speech as physiological limitations will allow.
2. Emphasize movement sequences.
3. Use task continua generated according to phonetic principles
4. Limit number of stimuli.
5. Use intensive, systematic drill.
6. Use the visual modality.
7. Facilitate response adequacy with systematic use of rhythm, intonation, stress, and motor movements.

speech system to preclude the facilitation of "normal" speech, even with extensive therapeutic efforts. Rosenbek and colleagues (1974) make an excellent point when they state: "Perhaps the reputation for poor prognosis inherited by these children reflects more on the speech pathologist's sometimes unrealistic goals than on these children's inability to communicate adequately" (p. 14). The authors also comment on the importance of this goal to "emphasize that apraxia is a volitional speech disorder and that language therapy and therapy to improve auditory discrimination and muscle strength are unnecessary unless deficits of language, discrimination or strength accompany the apraxia." (1974; p. 14). From the vantage point of many articles and studies that followed this 1974 paper, we now might want to reconsider at least a portion of this philosophy. Given the frequent, if not dominant, presence of expressive language deficits among developmental motor speech disorders (see Chapter 7), strong consideration for some form of language therapy should be included in most cases. This is not to condemn the position taken by Rosenbek and his colleagues, but rather to temper their position with the reality of later clinical and research findings.

Movement Sequences and Phonetic Principles

The next two items on the list of principles are closely related. This approach advocates emphasis on movement sequences during speech attempts and the selection of stimuli based on phonetic principles. Clinicians are advised not to focus on individual sounds, but to begin building speech-movement sequences from the CV or VC level, reduplicate these syllables (CVCV, etc.), and then systematically vary the consonants and vowels chosen as stimuli based coarticulatory principles similar to those described by McDonald (1964).

Do Not Overtax the System

Principles 4 and 5 also reflect a common underlying strategy: Do not overtax the information processing capabilities of the child. Limit the number of different stimuli being targeted and offer multiple, repetitive exposures to the same stimuli. They also advocate spacing or, more to the point, pacing the treatment session to avoid overloading the child.

Visual Versus Auditory Cues

The next principle directs clinicians to emphasize the visual modality in therapy and implicates a lesser role for auditory-based therapies. This position implies an auditory deficit as a component of developmental apraxia of speech. Although auditory processing deficits may be a components of these disorders (Crary, 1984a), the extent of these limitations and their potential influence of the speech-language deficits and on the selection of therapy strategies is virtually unknown. Another potential detriment of this advice is that clinicians may lean toward over-emphasis on the "visible sounds" of speech to the exclusion of the "invisible sounds" as therapy programs are structured. This situation reflects treating a label and its perceived philosophies rather than a child with a complex problem. There also are positive considerations for this principle. Many children will demonstrate improved performance in the presence of visual guidance or feedback. Others will benefit from multi-modality stimulation. Clinicians are encouraged to evaluate therapy techniques in reference to the potential influence of presentation in various modalities on the performance of the individual child.

Prosody and Gesture

The final principle on the advice list is to incorporate prosodic and/or gestural components into the therapy program. In younger children these might include rhymes, songs, and arm stress-timed movements. In older children written cues might be used to help the child modify the prosodic aspects of speech production.

Selective Application

Each of these principles advocated by Rosenbek et al. (1974) has potential value in designing and/or implementing a therapy program for some children with developmental motor speech disorders. Certain of the principles may apply to the dysarthric child as well as to children with various forms of apraxia of speech. Some of these principles would seem inappropriate for certain types of apraxic impairments. So, although there is value in each of these therapeutic principles, their limitations arise primarily from the authors' philosophy of the disorder to which they are applied. If, as suggested by the motolinguistic model, there are multiple forms of developmental motor speech disorders (including apraxias), then these principles would not be appropriate for all children. The clinician's task, then, becomes matching the performance profile to the therapeutic principle and selecting an appropriate treatment technique to achieve a specified goal.

Yoss and Darley (1974b)

Published back-to-back with the Rosenbek and colleagues' article was the perspective of Yoss and Darley (1974b). Actually, the Yoss and Darley article constitutes a review of previously published treatment philosophies regarding developmental apraxia of speech followed by a brief analysis of "commonly used therapy approaches." From this introduction they conclude by offering a list of nine suggestions for therapy in cases of developmental apraxia of speech. Table 9–2 summarizes their suggestions.

Building from the Bottom Up

These suggestions also delineate a bottom-up approach to therapy in cases of developmental apraxia of speech. In fact, six of the first seven items describe a step-by-step, building block format of a bottom-up intervention strategy. Initially, Yoss and Darley recommend nonspeech oral movement activities using a mirror for visual feedback. This step may be omitted for children who do not demonstrate an oral apraxia (i.e., impaired nonspeech oral movements). The next step is to have the child imitate vowels with exaggerated lip and mandible movement. The recommendation for exaggerated mandibular movement is interesting in light of suggestions that the mandible may play an assistive role in lingual movement and articulation (see Chapter 5). Next, visible consonants are introduced into the therapy scheme in an imitation format. Once "established" these are combined with vowels to form CV or VC combinations. Diphthongs are paired with consonants to introduce stress and intonational patterns accentuated by visible movements of the articulators. Suggestion number five is actually a comment on input modalities. As did Rosenbek and company, Yoss and Darley believed that auditory approach-

---

Table 9–2. Nine suggestions for therapy in cases of developmental apraxia of speech recommended by Yoss and Darley (1974b).

1. Begin with mirror work and imitation of all kinds of tongue and lip movements.
2. Have the child imitate sustained vowels.
3. Have the child imitate visible consonants.
4. Use consonant-diphthong pairings to introduce stress and intonational patterns accompanied by visible movements to accentuate changes in the placement of the articulators.
5. Visual input alone or paired with auditory stimuli leads to greater gains.
6. Move on to imitation of CVC shapes.
7. Extend sequencing efforts by using carrier phrases.
8. Facilitate self-monitoring often necessitating slower rate of speech.
9. Let the child's behavior provide the cues to what works best.

es (specifically, auditory discrimination) in isolation were of little benefit. They preferred emphasis on visual input, alone or in combination with auditory input. Item number six brings us back to the next step in the bottom-up hierarchy. Closed syllables (CVC) are introduced. The authors advocate use of rhyming words (real or nonsense) in minimal pairs. Finally, in suggestion (step) seven, sequencing efforts are extended by introducing a carrier phrase. Consonant clusters also are introduced at this point. Suggestions eight and nine are similar in nature to suggestion number five. They describe components that apply to all steps in the therapy program. Suggestion number eight advocates facilitation of self-monitoring of spontaneous speech as early as possible. Picture description or conversation are suggested techniques. This may necessitate slowing of speech rate by the child. The final suggestion seems to be a recommendation for an eclectic approach to treatment—let the child's behavior be your guide. If a given step or technique isn't appropriate, the child's performance may be a good indicator!

Teach Your Children Well

There is an additional aspect from the Yoss and Darley (1974b) article that merits consideration. In describing "therapy approaches used by school clinicians," these authors compared speech performances of 10 children following a 12- to 16-month interval of therapy. Each of these children appeared to have been "therapized" with some variant of a bottom-up treatment approach. Each made significant progress in speech tasks that would be considered to be at the bottom of the hierarchy described by Rosenbek et al. (1974) and by Yoss and Darley (1974b). According to Yoss and Darley (1974b), "it was apparent that articulation had significantly improved in terms of error rates for single words in repeated speech tasks" (p. 28). Even for two of the children who were judged clinically to be less intelligible on the follow-up speech sample, "in terms of correct production of phonemes in single words on repeated speech tasks, they showed significant improvement" (p. 28). Unfortunately, this was not a controlled study in which therapy techniques were systematically applied. Yet, from the information presented by Yoss and Darley, it seems apparent that the children involved had learned what had been presented to them: appropriate imitation of sounds in single words. The implication of this observation is that such children may perform well in speech-language therapy contrary to traditional opinion. However, it may be the nature of the therapy rather than the abilities or inabilities of the child that determines outcome.

The two reports described here are frequently cited as references for those designing therapy programs for children with apraxia of speech. However, given the spurt of clinical research studies in the late 1970s and 1980s, it is probable that philosophies and practices about intervention have changed since these manuscripts were published. Two more recent reviews may be used as a check on changing philosophies.

Pannbacker (1988)

Pannbacker (1988) summarized management strategies for developmental apraxia of speech with consideration of documentation regarding the effectiveness of the techniques reviewed. She presented five therapy principles based on previously published articles that were applicable to developmental apraxia of speech. These are:

1. There is no universally recognized single management procedure.
2. Therapy principles for the adult and child with apraxia of speech are very similar.
3. Management procedures for apraxia, dysarthria, and functional articulation disorders are basically the same.
4. Therapeutic emphasis should be on motor speech and language difficulties.
5. Diagnosis of developmental apraxia of speech often is made based on the length and results of therapy.

These principles indicate that, despite 14 to 16 years of intervening clinical research, little had changed in the perception of developmental apraxia of speech or its clinical management. With the exception of the inclusion of a language emphasis as a therapy component, these management principles implicate a bottom-up approach to therapy for these children. The final principle reinforces the belief that such approaches are not highly efficacious and that frustrated clinicians are drawn to the apraxia label secondary to slow or limited progress. The treatment techniques reviewed by Pannbacker (1988) further reinforce the focus on bottom-up approaches. Table 9–3 includes

Table 9–3. Selective therapy approaches available for developmental apraxia of speech according to Pannbacker (1988).

Type of Therapy	General Effectiveness
Adapted Cueing Technique (ACT)	Generally untested
Audiometer Integration	Untested
Hierarchies, Movement Sequencing, Systematic Drill	Preliminary results: Efficacious
Melodic Intonation Therapy	Generally untested
Nonspeech	Generally untested
Prompts for Restructuring Oral Muscular Phonetic Targets (PROMPT)	Untested
Signed Target Phoneme (STP)	Generally untested
Total Communication	Preliminary results: Efficacious
Touch-Cue System	Untested

Pannbacker's summary of therapy approaches available for developmental apraxia of speech.

Manual Emphasis

It is interesting to note that 6 of the 10 approaches recommended by Pannbacker involve a "manual" component—either using signs or gestures or physical shaping of oral consonants and vowels with tactile cues on the child's face and neck. One technique, melodic intonation therapy, emphasizes prosodic features and typically incorporates a gesture or baton-movement component to facilitate performance of rhythmic patterns. The multitude of possible therapy avenues that are not included in this review speak loudly to the perceptions of developmental apraxia of speech. Although many of the techniques listed might incorporate an auditory component, few emphasize learning via the auditory channel. Pannbacker addressed this aspect of treatment by citing the Rosenbek and Wertz (1972) and Yoss and Darley (1974b) articles which suggested that auditory *discrimination* approaches are probably inappropriate in such cases. In short, with the exception of melodic intonation therapy, which will be addressed later in this chapter, each of the approaches considered by Pannbacker (1988) to be appropriate for developmental apraxia of speech reflect a "build it from the bottom" philosophy of therapy. Movements are shaped into sounds which are subsequently shaped into monosyllabic units followed by attempts to sequence syllables. Perceptions of developmental apraxia of speech and its clinical management seem to have changed little despite intervening clinical research.

Marquardt and Sussman (1991)

Marquardt and Sussman (1991) also implicated a unitary disorder in developmental apraxia of speech and compared and contrasted this disorder and its intervention to functional articulation disorders (also referred to as phonological disorders). In reviewing a variety of therapy techniques ranging from phonetic placement to phonological rule-based procedures, Marquardt and Sussman (1991) suggested that "treatment regimens for DAS (developmental apraxia of speech) are based primarily on approaches developed for children with phonological disorders" (p. 358). This position seems to reflect a shift from the more traditional perspectives which are based to a large degree on principles applied to adults with apraxia of speech. However, there is more historical similarity than distinction in their recommended strategies.

Goals and Strategies

According to Marquardt and Sussman (1991), the "primary goals of treatment are to establish the complex, volitional sensorimotor production patterns that the child has failed to develop" (p. 358). Toward this end, they suggest that *treatment strategies for the apraxic child are distinguished by the use of cues, preferably visual and tactile cues, that assist in establishing movement patterns.* They advocate intensive, systematic drill to provide practice for these motor patterns. Isolated sounds are introduced initially in their treatment approach, typically vowels or consonants that are seen early in normal development or are highly visible. Subsequently, these sounds are presented in sequences forming nonsense syllables which are reduplicated and gradually shaped into meaningful words. Marquardt and Sussman recognize the appropriateness of other treatment approaches in cases of developmental apraxia of speech. They acknowledge the commentary of Rosenbek and Wertz (1972) who suggested that older children might address longer units of speech such as words and phrases rather than individual sounds. They also consider the positions of Crary (1984b) who advocated different treatment approaches based on performance profiles and Ekelman and Aram (1984) who advocated the inclusion of language deficits in treatment programs for the apraxic child. However, their basic position is distinctly bottom-up. This position derives from the conceptualization of developmental apraxia of speech as a unitary disorder.

Adapted Therapy Approaches

Like Pannbacker (1988), Marquardt and Sussman (1991) review what they refer to as "adapted therapy approaches" for developmental apraxia of speech. These include *PROMPT* (Chumpelik, 1984), *Touch-Cue* (Bashir, Graham-jones, & Bostwick, 1984) and *Melodic Intonation Therapy* (MIT) (Helfrich-Miller, 1984). According to Marquardt and Sussman (1991), these techniques incorporate therapy principles important to remediation in cases of developmental apraxia of speech. Both PROMPT and Touch-Cue rely primarily on tactile cues to facilitate movement patterns associated with speech sounds. MIT focuses on prosodic aspects of speech to facilitate improved speech production. As adapted by Helfrich-Miller (1984) for apraxic children, however, MIT incorporates the visual cues of sign language as well as attention to morphological and syntactic aspects of spoken language. Each of these specific techniques is presented in detail in Aram (1984).

Eight Treatment Principles—Revisited

Although oriented toward a specific, unitary concept of developmental apraxia of speech, the Marquardt and Sussman (1991) review includes many suggestions for treatment options. There is a subtle difference between their conceptualization of treatment approaches and prior positions. However, the similarities are much stronger than the differences. They offer sage advice in stating that "it is not possible to create a fail-safe cookbook for providing appropriate and efficient treatment for the child with DAS" (p. 365). In reviewing techniques they believe appropriate for these children, Marquardt and Sussman offer a set of eight treatment principles, which are summarized in Table 9–4. Compare this list of recommendations to those presented in Table

9–1 (Rosenbek et al., 1974) and 9–2 (Yoss & Darley, 1974b). It is apparent that more similarities than differences exist despite an extensive time span. This observation indicates that the essential perceptions of developmental apraxia of speech and its treatment had changed little over nearly a 20-year span. Since the publications of Rosenbek and Yoss were based in large part on the writings of Morley and others from the 1960s, it may be accurate to claim that little has changed in the perceptions of developmental apraxia of speech and its treatment for nearly 30 years. If these treatment strategies were highly successful, lack of change would be an acceptable clinical scenario. Unfortunately, this has not been the case.

A New Perspective: The Motolinguistic Model

A Conceptual Road Map

The model conceptualizing developmental motor speech disorders presented in this book incorporates most, if not all, of the traditional perspectives on developmental apraxia of speech, but expands those concepts to include congenital suprabulbar paresis and various forms of apraxic impairment. This model portrays a continuum of motor speech disorders in children rather than a unitary disorder commonly referred to as developmental apraxia of speech. Inherent in this conceptualization is the position that different forms of developmental motor speech disorders merit different treatment approaches. Perhaps the traditional reports of prolonged or failed therapy in cases of developmental apraxia of speech relate, in part, to a mismatch between the

Table 9–4. Eight principles for treatment of developmental apraxia of speech recommended by Marquardt and Sussman (1991).

1. Use of developmental norms for determining the sequence of speech sounds to be taught.

2. Maximum utilization of multimodal inputs (auditory, visual, tactual) to build articulatory movement patterns.

3. Recognition of facilitating effects of context in establishing target production.

4. Early introduction of self-monitoring skills to facilitate self-correction.

5. Intensive, systematic drill that provides repetition of sound patterns.

6. Emphasis on facilitatory effects of rhythm, stress, intonation, and motor activity in the production of sequences of speech sounds.

7. A hierarchical sequence of treatments proceeding from relatively simple canonical forms to more complex sequences with greater emphasis on movement sequences and syllabic integrity than on production of individual speech sounds.

8. Recognition of the necessity for guiding treatment based on the child's entry-level skills and responsiveness to different treatment approaches.

child's performance capabilities and the nature of the therapy program. The motolinguistic model provides a conceptual focus bridging assessment and treatment of the child with a suspected developmental motor speech disorder. By profiling performance abilities in different areas, it is possible to place a child toward one or the other end of the continuum. In a similar fashion, by analyzing the components of a treatment program, it is possible to place that program at one or the other end of the continuum. Some programs have a distinctly executive focus; others have a distinctly planning focus. In selecting a treatment program, it may be helpful to consider the components of the program in reference to the model and to the child. Essentially, the model becomes a conceptual road map that may help clinicians select more appropriate and hence efficacious treatment programs in cases of developmental motor speech disorders.

Analyzing a Treatment Program

Executive Programs

Executive deficits are characterized by difficulty with individual movements, sounds, and so on. Executive therapy programs focus on individual movements, sounds, and so on. In evaluating a therapy program, clinicians might ask if the program has a motoric or phonetic basis, focusing on individual sounds or coarticulatory sound sequences and attempting to build a spoken phonology from the bottom-up. Historically, the majority of therapeutic approaches offered in reference to developmental apraxia of speech would be considered "executive."

Planning Programs

Conversely, planning deficits are characterized by difficulty with movement/ sound sequences with better performance of isolated movements and individual sounds. Therapy programs that focus on word, phrase, or sentence level productions, emphasize semantic/syntactic aspects of phonological productions, and attempt to facilitate improved speech production from the top-down are considered "planning."

Knowing the Difference

Sometimes the character of a therapy program is obvious. If the program advocates establishing nonspeech movement patterns followed by individual sound production associated with those patterns, it follows an executive approach to therapy. In all likelihood, such programs subsequently will introduce a planning component, usually in the form of carrier phrases for target words. However, the basic structure of the program, including structuring of treatment sessions, selection of stimuli, and development of hierarchies is executive in nature. The focus throughout such programs is on production of specific sounds in an increasing number of contexts. Some programs might have a chameleon nature. If, for example, a program advocated production of target consonants at the end of different "roots" (e.g., boo-m, bea-m, ba-m, etc.), this program is closer to an executive than a planning focus. In fact, the majority of programs aimed at improvement of speech articulation performance would be classified as executive in nature. Programs with a planning focus are fewer in number, do not focus on production of individual sounds, and draw heavily on language abilities to facilitate improvement in speech production. The following discussion reviews five types of therapy programs in reference to the motolinguistic model to provide clinical examples of the principles, processes, and evaluation of therapy programs.

Traditional Articulation Therapies

As discussed above, many of the strategies applied to children with developmental motor speech disorders are modifications of traditional articulation therapies. Common modifications include emphasis on visual and/or tactile cuing, either in addition to or in place of auditory cuing, and the inclusion of some prosodic component in the therapy program. Each of these strategies would be oriented toward the executive end of the motolinguistic continuum. Each has a distinctly bottom-up flavor. The program designed by Rosenbek, Hansen, Baughman, and Lemme (1974) for their subject Kathy is an example of an executive approach to therapy. Because this program frequently is cited as an example of how to develop a therapy program for a child with an apraxia of speech, it should be addressed in detail. Please refer to the principles of therapy presented by these authors described earlier (Table 9–1).

Kathy

Kathy was a 9-year-old who had received speech therapy for 6 years. She was in the second grade, having repeated the first; yet, psychological testing revealed normal intelligence. The severe speech deficit most certainly played an influential role in her social and academic situation. Articulation testing indicated that the majority of errors were inconsistent omissions and substitutions. The term "inconsistent" was not defined in reference to evaluation procedures. All sounds except palatal affricates and fricatives were stimulable (i.e., she could produce them with cues and prompts) in single syllables. Articulation at the single word level was superior to that in connected speech. She demonstrated a reduced sentence length, omitting many functor words and some verb forms. Receptive language abilities were superior to expressive abilities. She demonstrated motoric struggle (initiation difficulties and groping) during speech attempts. She demonstrated a nonverbal oral apraxia on a facial movement task.

From this description we learn much about Kathy. First, she demonstrated persistence and patience of biblical proportions. Six years of speech therapy is a long time, and Kathy's difficulties probably frustrated and taxed more than one qualified clinician. We also note that, despite normal intelligence, she had repeated one grade. It is tempting to speculate that her speech difficulties were the direct cause of this situation; however, the indirect relationship of the speech deficit to a more overt reading difficulty may have been a factor. The authors mention social as well as academic difficulties. Again, these are attributed to the speech disorder. The characterization of her articulation errors is an initial reflection of a bottom-up approach to intervention. An articulation test that evaluates individual sounds within single word responses was used to obtain a "sound inventory." Although there is apparent consideration of performance load factors, the focus from the onset is on performance of isolated sounds. Finally, Kathy demonstrated an expressive language deficit marked by omission of various grammatical categories. The role of her nonverbal oral apraxia seemed to be only to confirm the diagnosis of apraxia of speech.

Kathy's Treatment Program

In keeping with an executive approach to therapy, the authors developed an intervention program with the express purpose of improving speech articulation abilities. The focus of speech therapy was the /r/ family of sounds because these errors were frequent and inconsistent. Because Kathy was an older child who demonstrated an organized sound repertoire, the initial step in therapy was to modify her speaking style. Specifically, she was taught to slow her speech rate by prolonging vowels and continuant consonants, increasing inter-word and syllable pauses, and inserting a schwa into consonant clusters. This goal was attained via recitation of stereotyped phrases, counting, and other more "automatic" speech activities. Language aspects of Kathy's performance were addressed by systematically manipulating one element of each phrase, such as the verb or object. No other description of the language component of therapy was provided. These speech exercises were accompanied by gross motor gestures such as swinging the arm in a semicircle, tracing a pattern with a finger, or squeezing a bean bag to mark each syllable. Written symbols were used as a visual cuing system to focus Kathy's attention on use of the various compensatory/facilitatory techniques. The presence of a specific symbol under a syllable indicated an arm swing or the insertion of a schwa. This pacing approach seemed primary to the prosodic adjustments sought in Kathy's speech. These drills were repeated systematically over several sessions. Kathy was required to evaluate her performance from tape-recorded samples to facilitate self-awareness.

Once the prosodic alterations in Kathy's speech were achieved, emphasis was placed on correct articulation of the /r/ family of sounds. Therapy progressed from the monosyllabic to the polysyllabic to the phrase and sentence level using the techniques learned during the initial portion of therapy. Subsequently, the "chewing method" was introduced to further slow Kathy's rate of speech. She was instructed to "chew like a cow" as she spoke target sentences.

These procedures were effective in facilitating Kathy's ability to produce the /r/ family of sounds over 22 consecutive therapy sessions spanning 3 months. This improvement had a positive influence on her overall intelligibility.

An Executive Approach

Why would this approach be considered an executive approach to therapy? The answer to that question contains more than one component: (1) The focus was on the production of individual sounds rather than on the reorganization of production phonology; (2) The procedures emphasized motor control for speech production rather than language-based influence; and (3) The organization of the program was bottom-up. Because phrases and sentences were employed as part of the program and language parameters were manipulated, it is tempting to postulate a planning component to this program. However, the motolinguistic model indicates that planning parameters are closer to language processing than to motor speech processing (see Chapter 3). Because the phrases and sentences employed in this program were automatic carriers, they probably involved little language processing in the sense that generation of novel phrases and sentences incorporates. The manipulation of language elements (verbs and/or objects) may reflect a planning component in this therapy program or these strategies may indicate a performance load strategy. The distinction is whether there is an attempt to facilitate language expansion interactive with improved speech performance or to use existing language forms to enhance improved speech performance. In short, there is no indication that Kathy was learning new language forms, and there was no focus on language performance. The same techniques could easily incorporate a planning component, however, by including steps to integrate novel language stimuli at a nonautomatic level. Such a modification would add a focus on expressive language abilities that could be interactive with articulation/phonological goals.

This program deviates somewhat from the classic bottom-up executive approach in that it uses phrase and sentence carriers to introduce target syllables and words. Yet, this approach is still executive in nature—the focus is distinctly on motor speech elements. Therapy simply begins at a higher performance load level. The reason for this situation is implied by the authors. Kathy was an older child with extensive therapy experience who had an organized sound repertoire. One implication of this case report is that, in older children who fit this scenario, it may be important to "shake-up" their habitual speaking pattern prior to attempts at establishing a new one.

Tactile Cuing Programs

Executive Emphasis

In general, tactile cuing approaches reflect an executive approach to articulation therapy. Despite variations in specific techniques, tactile cuing approaches attempt to modify articulation patterns by changing movement patterns during speech attempts. Typically, these programs begin at the individual sound level, either in isolation or in monosyllables, and attempt to improve production of that sound in various contexts from the bottom-up.

One of the earliest tactile cuing methods was that described by Stinchfield and Young (1938; Young & Hawk, 1955). In this approach the clinician provides manual cues to the child's face, such as approximating the lips followed by a quick release to stimulate bilabial productions. These movements are paired with an auditory image of the target sound.

Touch-Cue

More recent approaches seem to be direct descendants of the moto-kinesthetic approach, although each would claim uniqueness. The Touch-Cue approach (Bashir, Grahamjones, & Bostwick, 1984) is "recommended for persons who demonstrate articulation deficits characterized by problems in phoneme sequencing and patterning" (p. 128). The authors claim that this approach is *not* a speech-sound treatment approach. However, it appears to reflect a bottom-up orientation to therapy and is strongly executive in orientation. Tactile cues have been developed for eight oral consonants. These cues are paired with visual (watch me) and auditory (listen to me) cues to elicit production of isolated consonants. Visual and auditory cues are faded and the oral consonant subsequently paired with a neutral vowel to form a CV syllable. A second consonant is introduced and alternating CV syllables become targeted. Next, different vowels are introduced with each consonant. CVC syllables are introduced and the cue-fading process is repeated. Tactile cues eventually are faded. The final steps of the program include introduction of varying stimuli (pictures, open-ended sentences), polysyllabic words, and multiword sequences.

This program follows a classic progression from the isolated sound to production of that sound in syllables, words, phrases, and sentences. Nothing could be closer to a bottom-up philosophy of therapy. Also, the emphasis on movement patterns, coarticulation, and alternating syllabic sequences has a distinct motoric flavor. If the tactile cues are removed from this program, there is little difference between it and the traditional hierarchical stimuli approaches to articulation therapy. Like most programs, there is a strong performance load component inherent to the Touch-Cue technique. Yet, there seems to be little of a planning component as described in this chapter and in Chapter 3. The authors do concede that this program may accompany language therapy, but it is not intended as a replacement for language therapies. Finally, no efficacy data are provided for the Touch-Cue technique. In this regard clinicians are left to their own judgment to determine when to apply this procedure.

Prompts for Restructuring Oral Muscular Phonetic Targets

PROMPT (Chumpelik, 1984) is another tactile cue method. Designed to treat cases of developmental apraxia of speech as a movement disorder, this technique "focuses its treatment on the programming aspects of motor control . . . . by actually imposing a target position or sequence on the child." (Chumpelik, 1984; p. 141). The system of tactile cues in this program is much more complex than that used in the Touch-Cue program, incorporating cues for each English phoneme (vowels included). Unlike the Touch-Cue program PROMPT does not designate a systematic hierarchy of targets or cues. Rather, according to Chumpelik (1984), "each child . . . uses differing strategies to reach a target position or sequence a series of targets" (p. 151). This position necessitates extensive clinical knowledge of the PROMPT system in addition to physiologic phonetics and implies a detailed level of analysis of the child's articulatory abilities. At one level of analysis, the PROMPT program is similar to the Touch-Cue program. Both use tactile cues to facilitate improved performance in speech articulation abilities. Touch-Cue is specifically organized as a bottom-up program, whereas PROMPT seems to avoid such rigid hierarchical organization. Nonetheless, both programs are executive in nature, focusing on the motoric aspects of speech articulation, and neither offers convincing evidence of success nor suggestions for appropriate application.

Melodic Intonation Therapy (MIT)

Original Intent

MIT was initially developed as a technique to improve speech performance in adults with apraxia of speech (Sparks, Helm, & Albert, 1974; Sparks & Holland, 1976). Prosodic aspects of speech are modified to draw on the facilitating potential of melodic aspects of speech production. Patients learn stereotyped intonation, stress, and tempo patterns for the production of grammatically simple sentences accompanied by hand tapping. Clinician cues are gradually faded placing increasing responsibility on the patient for accurate performance.

Application to Children

MIT has received only limited attention concerning its application to children with apraxia of speech. Doszak, McNeil, and Jancosek (1981) applied these techniques as an experimental therapy to a 10-year-old boy judged to demonstrate an apraxia of speech. This boy demonstrated an established phonologic system with a substantial sound repertoire; however, he displayed many phonetic errors in conjunction with sound transpositions and substitutions. He had received traditional articulation therapy for 4 years with little improvement. This boy progressed through three target levels of the MIT program in two treatment sessions. Following this treatment, the authors concluded that the boy demonstrated significant reductions in vowel durations and the reduced perception of impaired speech. In short, for this child, MIT was a successful approach resulting in improved speech performance.

Schumacher, McNeil, and Yoder (1984) used the MIT approach experimentally with three children demonstrating apraxia of speech. Like the prior case study, these were older children ranging from 9½ years to 18 years, 9 months of age. This study evaluated target phoneme production at the monosyllable, bisyllable, phrase, and sentence levels within the MIT approach. Results indicated that each child made improvement in articulation of target phonemes at the respective levels in one to three sessions at each level. The authors concluded that, for the older children in this study, treatment at the monosyllable level was probably not necessary. However, unlike adults, the authors advised beginning at the bisyllable level rather than the phrase level.

Modifications Specific to Developmental Apraxia of Speech

Helfrich-Miller (1984) described a modification of the MIT approach specifically designed for cases of developmental apraxia of speech. She indicated that the ideal candidate for this approach is a child 7 to 8 years of age with a moderate to marked apraxia of speech. The child should demonstrate a mean length utterance of at least three to four words, poor repetition skills, and an attention span of 15 to 20 minutes. This adapted MIT program begins at the phrase level and progresses through three stages. The progression through these stages is characterized by increased phonologic and syntactic complexity of the target phrases. For example, phase I contains two- to three-word phrases which are grammatically simple and composed of vowels and bilabial stops. Phase II increases phrase length to four to five words with more complex consonants and grammatical morphemes. Phase III adds "maximum phonological, morphological, and syntactical complexity" (1984; p. 121). An interesting modification of the MIT approach is the replacement of hand tapping with Signed English. This was done in attempt to emphasize a language component to the MIT program. Helfrich-Miller reported successful outcomes in terms of articulation and phonemic sequencing abilities for two children during the MIT program, following the MIT program and at 6 month follow-up.

Executive, Planning, or Both

As described in these three reports, MIT may reflect either an executive or a planning approach to therapy. The MIT approach described in the first two reports (Doszak, et al., 1981; Schumacher, et al., 1984) seems to reflect an executive orientation to treatment. Very little phonologic or syntactic/semantic planning is represented in these more traditional MIT programs. The treatment strategy seems to be to modify the prosodic aspects of speech production toward the goal of enhancing performance of specific motor speech patterns associated with the production of consonants. There is a performance load component reflected in the progression from syllables to words to phrases to sentences, but this progression makes little effort to integrate linguistic planning aspects at any level. In this respect, the approach described in the first two reports is little different than the approach described by Rosenbek and his colleagues (1974) in which prosodic alteration is used to modify speech patterns toward the goal of improving production of individual speech sounds.

In contrast, the MIT approach described by Helfrich-Miller (1984) is more representative of a planning orientation to treatment. There is a focus on linguistic organization beginning at the phrase level with articulatory/phonologic complexity and syntactic complexity systematically increased as phrase length is increased. The use of manual sign language in substitution of hand tapping is a further reflection of a linguistic planning component is this modified approach.

Phonologic Approaches: Phonemic Contrasting

A Top-Down Approach: Semantics and Phonology

Marquardt and Sussman (1991) claim that treatment approaches for children with an apraxia of speech are based on approaches developed for children with phonological disorders. Yet, a recurring theme in this book is the presence of different types of phonological disorders. Many, if not most, of the traditional approaches to articulation therapy have an intrinsic executive orientation. The "phonological revolution" of the 1970s created a strong clinical emphasis on rule-governed phonological approaches to treatment. One of the prominent approaches emerging from this emphasis is phonemic contrasting. This approach has received extensive attention in published literature under a variety of labels including contrast therapy (Costello & Onstine, 1976) and minimal pairs orientation to distinctive feature training (Blache, 1978) in addition to phonemic contrast therapy (Fokes, 1982). Regardless of the label used and potential deviations in the specifics of the procedure among investigators and clinicians, the phonemic contrasting approach has a specific focus as a therapy program. The basic philosophy of this approach is to facilitate phonologic expansion by emphasizing semantic/syntactic distinctions that result from sound change. Stated succinctly by Blache (1978), "a speech sound is meant to *make words different*. That is what a phoneme is" (p. 272). The phonemic contrast procedure attempts to facilitate change in sound production by emphasizing semantic/syntactic distinctions between words differing by a single linguistic contrast. From this perspective, there are some important differences between this approach and traditional approaches. The unit of clinical focus is the meaningful word, not the sound or syllable. The focus is on phonological reorganization rather than motor speech execution; however, there is a strong "top-down" influence on the child to modify speech output to accommodate the linguistic distinctions inherent in the paired, contrasting stimuli. The message to the child is "if you want words to mean different things you must say them differently!". This top-down orientation represents a strong planning component to phonemic contrast therapy.

Components of Phonemic Contrasting

Though Blache (1978) takes a more theoretical, empirical approach to contrast therapy than Fokes (1982), both describe essentially the same components to the program. Phonemic contrast therapy incorporates many of the traditional components of therapy prescribed for the child with an apraxia of speech. Visual cues are utilized to establish the target contrast, there is structured and systematic repetition of the target contrast throughout the therapy session, and there is opportunity for building a performance load component into the program. Beyond these basics, Fokes (1982) advocates an interactive conversation based on a story told by the child using all of the stimuli targeted during the session. This addition represents an extension of the performance load component and emphasizes speech-language planning on the part of the child.

Linguistic Patterns Versus Individual Sounds

Because the focus of this approach is a linguistic contrast rather than a specific sound, clinicians may include multiple sounds in a therapy session. The correct production of the individual sound is a secondary consideration to evidence of the child's ability to somehow signal the linguistic contrast by changing speech patterns. Thus, for example, if a child was attempting to contrast CV versus CVC syllables, target pairs of stimuli might include "boy/boys," "go/goat" and "moo/moon." Initially, correct productions for the CVC words might include "boy/d/," "goa/d/," and "moo/d/" since the production of the contrastive element (CV vs. CVC) is more important than the production of the individual sound used to express that contrast. This emphasis reflects a major deviation from traditional, executive approaches in which the focus is on the correct production of individual sounds in various contexts.

Efficacy

Multiple reports have been offered highlighting the success of this treatment approach with children within the general category of phonological disorders, but none using phonemic contrasting as the sole treatment for speech improvement in cases of dysarthria or apraxia of speech in children. Crary and Hunt (1982) demonstrated that phonemic contrasting was a more efficient treatment approach than traditional articulation therapy (after Van Riper, 1972) in that it facilitated more improvement in a shorter amount of time. Weckler and Crary (1982) used phonemic contrasting as a component of a multifocal treatment program for three preschool-age boys considered to demonstrate an apraxia of speech. All three demonstrated substantial improvement in speech performance as a result of this intervention strategy. Although it is not possible to state unequivocally that the phonemic contrasting program was responsible for the observed changes, it appeared to play a significant role.

Language Therapies

A Lack of Emphasis

In general, language therapies have not been emphasized in reference to children with developmental motor speech disorders. Yet, the classic descriptions of dysarthric children with congenital suprabulbar paresis suggest that language deficits, especially expressive language deficits, are frequently seen. Also, there is ample evidence that children with apraxia of speech demonstrate significant expressive language deficits (see Chapter 7). In the intervention programs reviewed thus far, expressive language components are often touched on as a performance load component in therapy. That is, traditional programs direct the child to produce target sounds through a hierarchy of longer responses including sentences. Still, the modified MIT program described by Helfrich-Miller (1984) stands alone in advocating systematic introduction of grammatical complexity across the three hierarchical levels of the program. Finally, while phonemic contrasting approaches incorporate semantic/syntactic features, they do not address expressive language performance beyond the phonologic level.

Potential Targets

Included in her guidelines for treating children with apraxia of speech, Aram (Aram & Nation, 1982) recommends incorporation of semantic and syntactic goals, including vocabulary development, lexical retrieval, and syntax development. Ekelman and Aram (1984) documented that apraxic children receiving therapy did demonstrate improvement in syntactic expression. Their results and the results of Ekelman and Aram (1983) and Comeau and Crary (1982) may be used as preliminary guides in selecting targets of therapy aimed at improved syntactic expression. Of course, the selection of specific syntactic targets (or other language targets) will depend on the child's linguistic and conceptual abilities at that point in time. An obvious early goal of language therapy is the establishment of the closed (CVC) syllable. This step is deemed a necessary prerequisite or co-requisite to the introduction of morphophonemic markers. Either subsequent to, or in conjunction with this focus, Ekelman and Aram (1984) recommend that therapeutic efforts be directed to the syntactic areas listed in Table 9–5.

Strategic Plans

Experienced clinicians will realize immediately that many of these syntactic areas may be incorporated into a variety of therapy programs simply by selection of specific phrase and/or sentence stimuli. Also, many morphophonemic markers may be included directly into phonemic contrast approaches as stated above. Yet, these applications may not address directly the necessary levels of linguistic reorganization and performance load to facilitate improved syntactic expression. Ekelman and Aram (1984) offered their conceptualization of appropriate syntactic therapy strategies as follows:

Table 9–5. Eight syntactic areas requiring therapeutic intervention in cases of developmental apraxia of speech according to Ekelman and Aram (1984).

1. Copula and auxiliary "be" — first in declarative affirmative sentences and then in yes-no and wh-questions.
   Examples: "He is singing." "Is he singing?" "Why is he singing?"

2. Verb tenses, beginning with regular past, then future, then irregular past.
   Examples: "She played hard." "She will play hard." "She caught the ball."

3. Regular third person singular.
   Examples: "He talks." "She listens."

4. Pronouns — subjective, objective, and possessive forms.
   Examples: "she, he we, you, I"; "her, him, us, me"; "hers, his ours, your, my, mine."

5. Past participle -ed.
   Examples: "He has started." "She has finished."

6. Passive.
   Examples: "The ball was hit by the girl." "The boy was hit by the ball."

7. Yes-no and Wh-questions, stressing do-support and verb inversion.
   Examples: "Is it soup yet?" "When do we eat?"

8. Complex sentence constructions — conjunctions and embeddings.
   Examples: "The dog is barking and the man is yelling." "She got her coat because she was cold."

> Presentation of material toward the correction of these (syntactic) goals should be introduced visually. First, the child should "read" the new form, repeat the form with no visual cues, and then try to use the form in response to an auditory cue. When presenting new forms, the sentences should be short. As the new form becomes established, the sentence length may be elongated slowly. More complex sentence sequences are added and reinforced with selected use of pictures, scrambled sentences, and story completion techniques. Topics displaced in time and space are discussed and spontaneous spoken syntax corrected according to the syntactic form being worked on at the time. The primary goal of therapy is to teach the children syntactic structures that they can produce acceptably and intelligibly in conversational speech. (p. 108)

Many familiar concepts color this recommended therapy strategy. Similar to the traditional strategies recommended for articulation therapy in cases of developmental apraxia of speech described earlier, visual input is recommended. Novel forms are introduced in reduced performance load conditions. As performance improves, complexity is increased. Finally, the target is presented in a variety of contexts to facilitate learning to the point where it is used in natural conversation.

Weckler and Crary (1982) used many of these strategies in their multifocal treatment for developmental apraxia of speech. The expressive language component of their program relied heavily on the *Fokes Sentence Builder* (Fokes, 1976). In this technique, picture cards are used to represent words and syntactic markers. The child manually builds sentences by sequencing word-cards. The clinician controls the choice of targets and sentence length. By scrambling cards or turning them over, the clinician can introduce a performance load component focusing on sequencing skills and/or visual-verbal memory. Finally, the various sentences built during a therapy session may be used to facilitate an interactive storytelling component as an extension of performance load and planning functions.

Planning to the Extreme

Language therapy approaches would be considered to be at the extreme planning end of the motolinguistic continuum. Although many successful strategies for improving spoken language performance are available, the visual, sequencing aspects of the *Fokes Sentence Builder* or techniques that contain similar components may be most appropriate when language therapy is indicated in cases of development motor speech disorders.

Matching a Treatment Program to the Child

Clinical Profiling and the Motolinguistic Model

Selecting an appropriate treatment program is a crucial component of any intervention attempt. Not only must clinicians acquire an understanding of the difficulties and strengths demonstrated by a given child, they also must possess an understanding of the characteristics of potentially appropriate treatment programs. Clinical profiling following guidelines set forth by a model may be helpful in matching the program to the identified strengths and weaknesses displayed by the child. The motolinguistic model evaluates motor, speech, and language performances on a continuum from executive to planning. Treatment programs are evaluated from the same perspective. Thus, in a simple sense, it would seem appropriate to apply executive treatment programs to children demonstrating executive clinical performance profiles and planning treatment programs to children demonstrating planning clinical performance profiles. In many instances this will prove to be an effective intervention strategy. For example, the dysarthric child may require basic sensorimotor approaches to therapy along with techniques that alter the existing motor speech pattern prosodically (Stark, 1985; Yorkston, Beukelman, & Bell, 1988). Many of the motoric, bottom-up, executive articulation therapies would be appropriate in such cases. The same therapies have been recommended for use in cases of developmental apraxia of speech. The reason for this recommendation may be that the executive forms of apraxia, often those with the most overt motor symptoms, historically have been the focus for this label. The motolinguistic model places dysarthria close to executive forms of apraxia on the performance continuum. It should come as no surprise then that similar therapies would be appropriate in both instances.

On the other end of the continuum are the more linguistic, top-down, planning therapies. The overt recommendation would be to apply these strategies in cases where a planning performance profile is identified. However, planning interventions may have a more widespread application. Historically, two clinical scenarios are frequently encountered pertaining to children with developmental motor speech disorders: (1) Sounds may be produced in isolation and perhaps certain syllables and/or words, but without *carryover* into the more natural, conversational aspects of speech production; (2) Following years of treatment, speech production may be improved, but there is a remaining expressive language deficit. A single, as yet unanswered question, is pertinent to both of these observations. Are these "outcomes" the result of some intrinsic characteristic of the respective disorders or are they the result of misdirected treatment strategies? Yoss and Darley (1974b) reported that apraxic children did improve in their ability to produce isolated sounds in repetition tasks following what might be best described as a variety of executive therapies. Ekelman and Aram (1984) reported that apraxic children did demonstrate improvement in syntactic expression following speech-language therapy. It seems apparent then that children with developmental motor speech disorders are capable of learning—they learn what they are taught. If a therapy program emphasizes performance of oral movement patterns and production of isolated sounds in confined tasks, in all probability the child will demonstrate improved skills in these areas. If that program ignores the presence of an expressive language deficit, expectations of improvement in expressive language performance are unrealistic. The point of this monologue focuses on younger children with developmental motor speech disorders. Children do not learn spoken language systems one sound at a time. Language learning (including speech production aspects) incorporates a primary focus on integrative planning among a host of speech-language components. Therefore, for younger children, even those with a dysarthria or a severe executive form of apraxia of speech, clinicians must incorporate some planning, language component in the treatment plan. Older children who demonstrate a more advanced phonological system and expressive grammar may be better served by a focus on the executive components of intervention. This strategy is focused on improving intelligibility and maximizing the child's ability to use existing abilities. Children of any age who demonstrate a planning performance profile may be served best by treatment programs with a planning orientation. This strategy may reduce or eliminate the failure of therapy to establish carryover or to improve language expression. Finally, the very nature of developmental motor speech disorders calls for both an executive and a planning component in most, if not all, therapy programs. Clinicians should strive to establish a balance between executive and planning components dependent on the child's age, therapy history, and clinical performance profile. Table 9–6 summarizes these four strategic recommendations that should be useful when matching a treatment program to a child's clinical profile.

Table **9–6.** Four strategic recommendations for treatment planning in cases of developmental motor speech disorders.

1. In younger children, even those demonstrating a dysarthria or severe executive form of apraxia of speech, incorporate a significant planning, language component into the therapy program.

2. In older children demonstrating an executive performance profile (dysarthria or apraxia), executive treatment programs may prove more effective.

3. In children of any age demonstrating a planning performance profile, planning treatment programs may prove most effective.

4. In all cases of developmental motor speech disorders, treatment should incorporate a controlled balance between executive and planning therapies. The nature of that balance is determined by the child's age, prior therapy experience, and clinical performance profile.

Adjunctive Therapies

There Is a Need to Be Flexible

Nature has organization. Unfortunately, sometimes we have difficulty identifying the nature of that organization. Clinicians should be wary of any strategy that claims to be a panacea. The recommendations based on the motolinguistic model are *only* recommendations, they are not prescriptive. Instances will occur during which clinicians will encounter difficulties in children with developmental motor speech disorders that require interventions beyond those implicated in this chapter. Recall from Chapter 1 that Worster-Drought (1974) described drooling, dysphagia, and velopharyngeal dysfunction as frequent deficits among children with congenital suprabulbar paresis. Rosenbek and Wertz (1972) identified drooling and feeding problems among their group of children with apraxia of speech. Others have reported that some children with apraxia of speech may not speak at all (Ferry, Hall, & Hicks, 1975). Too, there may be instances in which the motor speech dysfunction is so severe that the prognosis for functional speech production is limited. Clinical intervention in these cases often incorporates what might be termed adjunctive therapies. Fortunately, these are not the majority of cases encountered among children with developmental motor speech disorders. When such situations are encountered, however, they often represent the most severe deficits and the greatest clinical challenges.

Types of Adjunctive Interventions

Adjunctive therapies may be designed to restore lost functions, compensate for severely impaired functions, serve as a transitional facilitator to develop a function, or improve functions related to speech performance. These therapies are not specific to developmental motor speech disorders, but may be appropriate, even required, in certain cases. The child with velopharyngeal deficits may require surgery or a prosthesis to improve speech function (Hall, Hardy, & LaVelle, 1990; Stark, 1985; Yorkston, Beukelman, & Bell, 1988). Some children may benefit from alternative-augmentative communication systems either in replacement for speech functions or to facilitate improvement in verbal output. Others may benefit from computer-interactive and assisted strategies either to augment communication functions or to facilitate communicative learning. Jaffe (1984) recommended extensive use of sign language strategies to facilitate increased verbalizations and meaningful gestures in children with apraxia of speech. Other possibilities might include using pictures of highly motivating items (cookies, juice, etc) placed strategically around the home as a method to facilitate interactive communication between child and parent. Such strategies may increase verbal attempts by the non-speaking or minimally verbal child. The clinical management of feeding and swallowing difficulties also may be relevant in certain types of developmental motor speech disorders. Such difficulties may require surgical, medical, and/or behavioral therapies. The important point is that clinicians should be aware of the potential for these deficits to occur among children with developmental motor speech disorders. In cases where such deficits are prominent, it may be necessary to address them prior to or in conjunction with other forms of intervention.

A Multifocal Intervention Program

Throughout this book there has been an emphasis on motor, motor speech, phonologic, and grammatic aspects of speech-language performance among children demonstrating a developmental motor speech disorder. At best, most of the above-mentioned therapies address only one or two of these elements. Weckler and Crary (1982) proposed a multifocal therapy program designed for children with an apraxia of speech. This program was not developed in reference to the motolinguistic model, but in response to the dominant trilogy of motor speech, phonologic, and syntactic deficits frequently seen in children with an apraxia of speech. The program contains three phases representing the motor speech, phonologic, and syntactic areas of deficit seen in these children. All three phases are intended to be addressed in each therapy session rather than in a hierarchical fashion as recommended traditionally. Following is a description of this program with a retrospective comparison of each phase to the motolinguistic model. A sample program is presented in Appendix F.

Phase I: Motor Speech

Purpose

The initial phase is intended as a series of oral motor phonetic drills. This phase is highly executive in nature, building on phonetic principles and increasing the performance load factor systematically. The goal of this phase is to improve independent lingual movement during speech. Recall from Chapter 5 that many children with developmental apraxia of speech may demonstrate a lingual-mandibular dependency. Using a bite block to stabilize the mandible and reduce mandibular support during speech may help to increase independent lingual movement and result in improved oral articulation for speech. This technique was incorporated into more traditional articulation drills as the initial phase of the program.

Procedure

A bite block is placed between the first molars on one or both sides, depending on the child's degree of tolerance. With the block in place and following a period in which the child adjusts to the presence of the block, a series of speech sounds and sound sequences are presented for imitation by the child. The three vowels of the "vowel triangle" (/i/, /a/, and /u/) are presented first. These sounds were chosen because they facilitate maximum movement of the tongue within the oral cavity in a nonconsonant context. These isolated vowels were followed by vowel-vowel sequences, vowel-glide-vowel sequences, and vowel-obstruent or obstruent-vowel sequences. The number of syllables in the sequences was increased gradually as the child's performance improved at each level. Different coarticulatory combinations were used to facilitate the goal of improved independent lingual movement during speech attempts. Finally, CVC syllables and syllable sequences were introduced. This phase typically is difficult for the child to tolerate and is limited to 5 to 10 minutes at the beginning of each treatment session. It is important to note that the goal of this phase was to provide an environment that facilitates maximum independent lingual movement during speech. In this respect, the correct production of the sounds used is secondary to the clinician's observation of appropriate lingual movement.

Phase II: Phonological Reorganization

Purpose

The purpose of the second phase was to improve the child's phonological performance. The phonemic contrasting approach, identified above as a planning strategy, was used. The rationale for this approach was to use one of the child's strength areas (semantic knowledge) to facilitate improvement in a major deficit area (phonological performance).

Procedure

Phonemic contrasting consists of four major components: (1) modeling, (2) discrimination, (3) production, and (4) performance load building (Blache,

1982; Fokes, 1982). Pictures are prepared for each minimal word-pair. These pictures are presented to the child along with a spoken model. At this time, the contrast is made obvious to the child in two ways. The clinician may use a visual display containing pockets identified with pictures depicting the contrast feature. Each word in the pair is spoken, identified with one feature of the contrast, and placed in the appropriate pocket. For example, if the contrast is "open-closed" syllables (words), a suitable word-pair might be "boo" and "boom." The clinician presents one word (boo), identifies the contrast feature (boo is an open word), and places the picture in the appropriate pocket (pocket with picture of open mouth). Subsequently, the clinician presents the other word (boom), identifies the contrast feature (boom is a closed word), and places the picture in the appropriate pocket (pocket with picture of closed mouth). Initially, especially for younger children, it may be helpful if the clinician exaggerates the contrast feature (i.e., prolongs the vowel of the open word and/or shortens the vowel of the closed word and prolongs the final consonant, if possible). All word-pairs are presented (modeled) before progressing to the next step.

The second step evaluates the child's ability to hear the contrast distinction in the various word-pairs. The paired pictures are presented, one pair at a time, and the clinician names one of the words. The child is requested to identify the picture named and to put that picture in the appropriate pocket. This step is helpful in determining whether the child can discriminate the distinctions and how well the child has learned the contrast analogy presented in the first step.

Blache (1982) refers to step three as "the moment of truth." At this juncture the clinician and child reverse roles and the child names the pictures. The clinician must be careful to select the picture actually named by the child, even if it is clear that the other picture was the target. It is at this step that the true meaning of "the pragmatic phoneme" is revealed to the child. In the certain event of failure on one or more of the attempts, the clinician may use a variety of strategies to facilitate an appropriate production. Fokes (1982) takes a more pragmatic approach requesting a repair via interactive conversation. Weckler and Crary (1982) used an intervening imitation step between discrimination and production. An important point is to not drill the individual word productions. Rather, move on to the next word pair.

The final step in this technique is performance load building. Several strategies may be applied here. The most immediate technique is to place all of the pictured words into a pile and ask the child to retrieve them one at a time. As the cards are retrieved, the child, with or without assistance from the clinician, tells a story using all of the words. The clinician may use this opportunity to request repairs, ask for expansions, or otherwise attempt to incorporate the word productions into longer phrase and sentence units. This phase of the multifocal program may be completed in approximately 20 minutes.

Phase III: Syntactic Performance

Purpose

The final phase of the program is designed to improve syntactic expression and to serve as a carryover step for the phonological targets presented in the second phase.

Procedure

Clinicians may employ any number of therapy techniques during this phase; however, the *Fokes Sentence Builder* or similar techniques emphasizing visual and sequencing components may be especially appropriate for the child with an apraxia of speech. The word-pairs used in phase II are incorporated into this phase of the program. Thus, during this activity, the clinician has the opportunity to address phonological performance as well as syntactic expression. Experience suggests that only a single novel element be introduced at one time. For example, if a new phonological contrast or new word-pair for an existing contrast is introduced during a session, it should be presented in the context of an established syntactic target. New syntactic targets should be presented in the context of established phonologic contrasts and known word-pairs. This strategy may be referred to as "stair stepping." In other words, only a single novel element is introduced during a particular treatment session. Once this element is established, it remains constant while a different novel element is introduced. The two elements at this stage are phonologic and syntactic performance. Similar to phase II, this aspect of the program should be ended in a storytelling or conversational mode.

Efficacy of the Multifocal Program

Weckler and Crary (1982) reported progress noted in three boys with an apraxia of speech between the ages of 4 and 5 years over a 6-week period of therapy. These boys were seen 3 days each week for 45-minute individual treatment sessions. One of the boys received therapy using the multifocal program for all 6 weeks, one for 5 of the 6 weeks and one for 4 of the 6 weeks. Sessions not incorporating the program were interactive play sessions used for baseline data recording.

Short-Term Benefits

The results of diadochokinetic, phonologic, and syntactic performances at the end of the 6 week period indicated that each of the boys progressed in each area. Syntactic change reflected the grammatical frames targeted in the treatment programs. Phonologic change reflected the targeted error patterns but also revealed other changes suggestive of some degree of phonological reorganization. Change in diadochokinetic performance was not dramatic but was noted for the two boys receiving 6 and 5 weeks of therapy. The child receiving 4 weeks of therapy demonstrated no change on the diadochokinetic measure. Furthermore, there seemed to be some correlation between phonologic change and change on diadochokinetic performance. The boy receiving the most treatment demonstrated the most change on these measures, followed by the boy receiving the second largest amount of treatment, followed by the boy receiving the least treatment. These initial results suggested that the multifocal program has the potential to produce motor-speech, phonologic and syntactic change in as little as 4 to 6 weeks of treatment. This short duration of treatment was insufficient to bring the children's performances within acceptable limits, but substantial change was produced in a relatively short time.

Benefits from Extended Treatment

Malinsky (1985) was able to continue treatment sessions for two of the three boys for an extended period of time. The two boys receiving the most therapy in the initial study received additional therapy for 18 and 7 months, respectively. Each of these boys continued to progress relative to phonologic and syntactic performance. At the end of the program both boys were intelligible and produced near age-appropriate scores on standard articulation tests. They also demonstrated improved syntactic expression with utterance lengths averaging nearly six morphemes and the emergence of complex sentence structures. The child who received the most initial therapy required some additional treatment addressing prosodic aspects of speech and syntactic expression. The second child was dismissed from therapy at that time.

The collective result of these two reports is that the multifocal program has the potential to produce change in speech-language performances in a relatively short period of time and may be an effective strategy to bring these performances into acceptable ranges. Malinsky (1985) did note that the program was enhanced in the later stages primarily to increase each boy's self-awareness of performance in interactive conversation. She emphasized pragmatic techniques and parent involvement to facilitate self-awareness in the later stages of treatment. This strategy is consistent with traditional approaches to therapy in cases of developmental apraxia of speech as presented earlier in this chapter.

Application of the Multifocal Program

The multifocal program contains elements with both an executive and a planning focus. Furthermore, it addresses the three primary areas of deficit associated with developmental motor speech disorders. This program may be applicable to many children with developmental motor speech disorders including dysarthria, executive forms of apraxia, and planning forms of apraxia. An obvious strategy would be to manipulate the balance among the three components of the program to fit the clinical performance profile of the child.

A dysarthric child with a significant oromotor deficit and speech articulation errors associated with specific aspects of this deficit may require much more attention at the first phase of the program than the second phase. Yet, since these children, especially at a younger age, may demonstrate disrupted phonological organization and syntactic expression, some attention to these aspects might well be included in each therapy session. A similar strategy may be applied to the child with a severe executive form of apraxia of speech. Conversely, the child demonstrating a planning form of apraxia of speech may require little or no focus on the motor-speech components of the first phase of the program. In short, the multifocal program was designed as a flexible strategy rather than a hierarchical prescription.

Some Final Comments on Intervention Strategies

Clinicians should be aware that precious little research has been completed on the effectiveness of intervention strategies applied to children with developmental motor speech disorders. Part of the responsibility for this absence of treatment efficacy research lies with the absence of a conceptual framework surrounding developmental motor speech disorders. The motolinguistic model offers such a conceptual framework. If the mystery of inefficient treatment in these cases is to be solved, systematic clinical trials must be applied to children grouped on the basis of common clinical performance profiles.

None of the intervention strategies, programs, or techniques just discussed can lay claim to being *the* treatment for children with developmental motor speech disorders. However, each and every one of them *may* be appropriate in a given case. Intervention begins with the clinician's perceptions of the problem. Clinical assessment and treatment strategies often are driven by the clinician's perceptions of the underlying problem. If the problem is perceived solely as a motor problem, the intervention probably will pursue strategies to improve motor functions pertaining to speech production. If the problem is perceived as a phonologic and/or language problem, different strategies will be implemented. The motolinguistic model offered in this book provides a perspective on developmental motor speech disorders that is broader than traditional concepts. It advocates a multifocal perspective on developmental motor speech disorders that influences both the clinical evaluation and the selection and implementation of intervention strategies. This model is not a panacea, but rather an alternative. It should be viewed as such.

Clinically Relevant Highlights

Developmental motor speech disorders are defined as a *group* of disorders rather than a unitary speech problem. Intervention in these cases must recognize and adjust for the diversity of potential problems encountered in individual children. The philosophy of treatment proffered by the motolinguistic model is based on selecting treatment strategies matched to the abilities of the child. In characterizing treatment approaches, a few "rules of thumb" may help.

1. Executive treatment approaches emphasize motoric, phonetic aspects of speech production and attempt to build speech and language performance from the bottom up.

2. Planning treatment approaches emphasize linguistic organization (phonological, syntactic, semantic) and attempt to stimulate improved speech performance from the top down.

3. Instances will be encountered in which adjunctive therapies are indicated, either to facilitate improved speech performance or to establish functional, interactive communication.

4. **Many cases of developmental motor speech disorders will reveal a mix of executive and planning deficits; therefore, treatment approaches should include a mix of strategies. A multifocal intervention framework is offered as an example of this approach.**

Experienced clinicians will recognize many, if not most, of the individual treatment techniques discussed in this chapter. Technique is not the key issue, perspective is. By addressing multiple components of multidimensional problems in a systematic manner, the probabilities for successful intervention are enhanced. The motolinguistic model does not offer answers, it offers direction. Sometimes the direction will be a short cut to success. Sometimes it will be a long and winding road. There is little doubt, however, that elements of the model, applied judiciously and creatively, can facilitate an improved quality to communicative life for children who struggle with words.

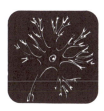

Epilogue

Warm Feelings

Dear Doctor

Thanks so much for your help with my son. His clinician has been using the approach you suggested for the last month and we are seeing changes already. He is less frustrated now when he tries to tell us things. And, we really do understand him better. He spoke to his grandmother on the phone last weekend and she could understand him. We realize that there is a long way to go, but this is the most positive change we have seen in a long time. Our heartfelt thanks.

Sincerely,

Leonard's Mom

Letter's like this one should be more commonplace. The information in this book will help some clinicians help some children. Large gaps in information exist and the difficulties of some children are beyond the scope of this book. It is (sometimes painfully) apparent that historical, traditional approaches to assessment and intervention in cases of developmental motor speech disorders do not produce the desired outcomes in too many cases. Rather than throw out the baby with the bathwater, a different perspective may help clinicians to focus their efforts in a different direction. As the line from a song by Jimmy Buffett goes: "Forget that blind ambition and trust your intuition."

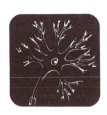

References

Albert, M., Goodglass, H., Helm, N., Rubens, A., & Alexander, M. (1981). *Clinical aspects of dysphasia.* New York: Springer-Verlag.

Altman, J. (1967). Postnatal growth and differentiation of the mammalian brain with implications for a morphological theory of memory. In C. Quarton, T. Melnechuk, & F. Schmitt (Eds.), *The neurosciences* (pp. 723–744). New York: Rockefeller University Press.

Aram, D. (1980, November). *What ever happened to functional articulation disorders?* Presentation at the American Speech-Language-Hearing Association Convention, Detroit, MI.

Aram, D. (1984). *Seminars in speech and language: Vol. 5. Assessment and treatment of developmental apraxia.* New York: Thieme-Stratton.

Aram, D., & Glasson, C. (1979, November). *Developmental apraxia of speech.* Miniseminar presentation at the American Speech-Language-Hearing Association Convention, Atlanta.

Aram, D., & Horwitz, S. (1983). Sequential and nonspeech praxic abilities in developmental verbal apraxia. *Developmental Medicine and Child Neurology, 25,* 197–206.

Aram, D., & Nation, J. (1975). Patterns of language behavior in children with developmental language disorders. *Journal of Speech and Hearing Research, 18,* 229–241.

Aram, D., & Nation, J. (1982). *Child language disorders.* St. Louis: C.V. Mosby.

Bashir, A., Grahamjones, F., & Bostwick, R. (1984). A touch-cue method of therapy for developmental verbal apraxia. *Seminars in Speech and Language, 5,* 127–137.

Baum, S., & Katz, W. (1988). Acoustic analysis of compensatory articulation in children. *Journal of the Acoustical Society of America, 84,* 1662–1668.

Bishop, S., & Edmundson, A. (1987). Language-impaired 4-year-olds: Distinguishing transient from persistent impairment. *Journal of Speech and Hearing Disorders, 52,* 156–174.

Blache, S. (1978). *The acquisition of distinctive features.* Baltimore: University Park Press.

Blache, S. (1982). Minimal words pairs and distinctive feature training. In M. Crary (Ed.), *Phonological intervention: Concepts and procedures* (pp. 61–96). San Diego: College-Hill Press.

Blakeley, R. (1980). *Screening test for developmental apraxia of speech.* Tigard, OR: C.C. Publications.

Bowman, S., Parsons, C., & Morris, D. (1984). Inconsistency of phonological errors in developmental verbal dyspraxic children as a factor of linguistic task and performance load. *Australian Journal of Human Communication Disorders, 12,* 109–119.

Brooks, V. B. (1986). *The neural basis of motor control.* New York: Oxford University Press.

Brown, J. (1979). Language representation in the brain. In H. Steklis & M. Raleigh (Eds.), *Neurobiology of social communication in primates: An evolutionary perspective* (pp. 133–195). New York: Academic Press.

Brown, J. K. (1985). Dysarthria in children—neurologic perspective. In J. K. Darby (Ed.), *Speech and language evaluation in neurology: Childhood disorders* (pp. 13–184). New York: Grune & Stratton.

Brown, R. (1973). *A first language.* Cambridge, MA: Harvard University Press.

Byring, R., & Pulliainen, V. (1984). Neurological and neuropsychological deficiencies in a group of older adolescents with dyslexia. *Developmental Medicine and Child Neurology 26,* 765–773.

Campbell, T. F., & McNeil, M. R. (1985). Effects of presentation rate and divided attention on auditory comprehension in children with an acquired language disorder. *Journal of Speech and Hearing Research, 28,* 513–520.

Cappa, S., Cavolotti, G., & Vignolo, L. (1981). Phonemic and lexical errors in fluent aphasia: Correlation with lesion site. *Neuropsychologia, 19,* 171–177.

Caramazza, A., Berndt, R., & Basili, A. (1983). The selective impairment of phonological processing: A case study. *Brian and Language, 18,* 128–174.

Catts. H. (1986). Speech production/phonological deficits in reading-disordered children. *Journal of Learning Disabilities, 19,* 504–508.

Catts, H. (1989). Speech production deficits in developmental dyslexia. *Journal of Speech and Hearing Research, 54,* 422–428.

Cermak, S. (1985). Developmental dyspraxia. In E. A. Roy (Ed.), *Neuropsychological studies of apraxia and related disorders* (pp. 225–248). North Amsterdam: Elsevier Science.

Chappell, G. (1973). Childhood verbal apraxia and its treatment. *Journal of Speech and Hearing Disorders, 38,* 362–368.

Chi, J. D., Dooling, E. C., & Gilles, F. H. (1977). Left-right asymmetries of the temporal speech areas of the human fetus. *Archives of Neurology, 34,* 346–348.

Chumpelik, D. (1984). The prompt system of therapy: Theoretical framework and applications for developmental apraxia of speech. *Seminars in Speech and Language, 5,* 139–156.

Colheart, M. (1980). Deep dyslexia: A review of the syndrome. In M. Colheart, K. Patterson, & J. C. Marshall (Eds.), *Deep dyslexia* (pp. 22–47). Boston: Routledge & Kegan Paul.

Comeau, S., & Crary, M. A. (1982, November). *Developmental verbal apraxia: A morphophonemic analysis*. Presentation at the American Speech-Language-Hearing Association Convention, Toronto.

Conel, J. L. (1939–1963). *Postnatal development of the human cerebral cortex* (Vols. 1–6). Cambridge, MA: Harvard University Press.

Costello, J., & Onstine, J. (1976). The modification of multiple articulation errors based on distinctive features theory. *Journal of Speech and Hearing Disorders, 42,* 199–215.

Crary, M. A. (1982, August). *Descriptive power of phonological analysis: Implications for assessment and therapy with unintelligible children*. Presentation at the Northcentral Regional Conference of the American Speech-Language-Hearing Association, Milwaukee.

Crary, M. A. (1984a). A neurolinguistic perspective on developmental verbal dyspraxia. *Communicative Disorders, 9,* 33–49.

Crary, M. A. (1984b). Phonological characteristics of developmental verbal dyspraxia. *Seminars in Speech and Language, 5,* 71–83.

Crary, M. A. (1991, November). *What have we learned about developmental apraxia of speech?* Miniseminar presentation to the American Speech-Language-Hearing Association, Seattle.

Crary, M. A., & Anderson, P. (1990, February). *Speech and nonspeech motor performance in children with suspected developmental dyspraxia of speech*. Presentation to the International Neuropsychological Society, Orlando, FL.

Crary, M. A., & Comeau, S. (1982, November). *Phonological process suppression in normal children*. Presentation at the American Speech-Language-Hearing Association, Toronto.

Crary, M. A., & Fokes, J. (1980). Phonological processes in apraxia of speech: A systematic simplification of articulatory performance. *Aphasia-Apraxia-Agnosia, 1,* 1–13.

Crary, M. A., Hardy, T., & Williams, W. (1985) Aphemia: With dysarthria or apraxia of speech? *Proceedings of the Cinical Aphasiology Conference.* Minneapolis: BRK Publishers.

Crary, M. A., & Hunt, T. L. (1982). Sounds vs patterns: A case comparison of approaches for articulation therapy. *Australian Journal of Human Communication Disorders, 10,* 15–22.

Crary, M. A., & Hunt, T. L. (1983). CV to CVC: A case report of a child with open syllables. *Topics in Language Disorders, 3,* 157–170.

Crary, M. A., Landess, S., & Towne, R. (1984). Phonological error patterns in developmental verbal dyspraxia. *Journal of Clinical Neuropsychology, 6,* 157–170.

Crary, M. A., & Towne, R. L. (1984). The asynergistic nature of developmental verbal dyspraxia. *Australian Journal of Human Communication Disorders, 12,* 27–38.

Crary, M. A., Towne, R. L., Comeau, S., & Korte, S. (1982, June). *Is verbal apraxia a phonological disorder?* Presentation at the Symposium on Research in Child Language Disorders. Madison, WI.

Crary, M. A., Turner, G., & Williams, W. (1990, November). *What do bite blocks do?* Presentation at the Speech-Language-Hearing Association, St. Louis.

Crary, M. A., Voeller, K. K. S., & Haak, N. J. (1988). Questions of developmental neurolinguistic assessment. In M. Tramontana & S. Hooper (Eds.), *Assessment issues in child neuropsychology* (pp. 249–279). New York: Plenum Press.

Crary, M. A., Welmers, T., & Blache, S. (1981, August). *A preliminary look at phonological process suppression.* Presentation at the Second International Congress for the Study of Child Language, Vancouver.

Crome, L. (1960). The brain and mental retardation. *British Medical Journal, 16,* 897–904.

Curtis, S. (1985). The development of human cerebral lateralization. In D. F. Benson & E. Zaidel (Eds.), *The dual brain: Hemispheric specialization in humans* (pp. 97–116). New York: Guilford Press.

Darley, F. (1969, November). *Aphasia: Input and output disturbances in speech and language processing.* Presentation at the American Speech and Hearing Association, Chicago.

Darley, F., Aronson, A., & Brown, J. (1975). *Motor speech disorders.* Philadelphia: W. B. Saunders.

De Renzi, E., Pieczuro, A., & Vignolo, L. (1966). Oral apraxia and aphasia. *Cortex, 2,* 50–73.

de Villiers, J., & de Villiers, P. (1973). A cross-sectional study of the acquisition of grammatical morphemes in child speech. *Journal of Psycholinguistic Research, 2,* 267–268.

DeJarnette, G. (1988). Formant frequencies (F1, F2) of jaw-free versus jaw-fixed vowels in normal and articulatory disordered children. *Perceptual and Motor Skills, 67,* 963–967.

Denckla, M. B. (1981). Minimal brain dysfunction and dyslexia: beyond diagnosis by exclusion. In M. Blaw, I. Rapin, & M. Kinsbourne (Eds.), *Child neurology* (pp. 243–262). New York: Spectrum.

Dennis, M., & Whitaker, H. (1976). Language acquisition following hemi-decortication: Linguistic superiority of the left over right hemisphere. *Brain and Language, 3,* 404–433.

Dewey, D., & Kaplan, B. J. (1992). Subtyping of developmental motor deficits. *Journal of Clinical and Experimental Neuropsychology, 14,* 50. (Abstract)

Dewey, D., Roy, E. A., Square-Storer, P., & Hayden, D. (1988). Limb and oral praxic abilities of children with verbal sequencing deficits. *Developmental Medicine and Child Neurology, 30,* 743–751.

DiSimoni, F. (1978). *The Token Test for Children.* Boston: Teaching Resources.

Dollaghan, C. A., Campbell, T. F., & Tomlin, R. (1990). Video narration as a language sampling context. *Journal of Speech and Hearing Disorders, 55,* 582–590.

Doszak, A., McNeil, M. R., & Jancosek, E. (1981, November). *Efficacy of melodic intonation therapy with developmental apraxia of speech.* Presentation at the American Speech-Language-Hearing Association Convention, Los Angeles.

Drake, W. E. (1968). Clinical and pathological findings in a child with developmental learning disabilities. *Journal of Learning Disabilities, 1,* 486–502.

Dworkin, J. (1978). A therapeutic technique for improvment of lingual alveolar valving abilities. *Language, Speech and Hearing Services in Schools, 9,* 169–175.

Dworkin, J., & Culatta, R. (1980). *Dworkin-Culatta oral mechanism examination (D-COME).* Nicholasville, KY: Edgewood Press.

Edwards, M. L., & Shriberg, L. (1983). *Phonology: Applications in communicative disorders.* San Diego: College-Hill Press.

Ekelman, B., & Aram, D. (1983). Syntactic findings in developmental verbal apraxia. *Journal of Communication Disorders, 16,* 237–250.

Ekelman, B., & Aram, D. (1984). Spoken syntax in children with developmental verbal apraxia. *Seminars in Speech and Language, 5,* 97–110.

Falzi, G., Perrone, P., & Vignolo, L. (1982). Right-left asymmetry in anterior speech region. *Archives of Neurology, 39,* 239–240.

Feinberg, T., Rothi, L., & Heilman, K.M. (1986). "Inner speech" in conduction aphasia. *Archives of Neurology, 43,* 591–593.

Ferry, P., Hall, S., & Hicks, J. (1975). "Dilapidated" speech: Developmental verbal dyspraxia. *Developmental Medicine and Child Neurology, 17,* 749–756.

Finger, S., & Stein, D. (1982). *Brain damage and recovery: Research and clinical perspectives.* New York: Academic Press.

Flechsig, P. (1901). Developmental (myelogenetic) localization of the cortex in human subjects. *Lancet, 2,* 1027–1029.

Fletcher, S. (1972). Time-by-count measurement of diadochokinetic syllable rate. *Journal of Speech and Hearing Research, 15,* 763–770.

Fokes, J. (1976). *Fokes sentence builder.* Hingham, MA: Teaching Resources.

Fokes, J. (1982). Problems confronting the theorist and practitioner in child phonology. In M. A. Crary (Ed.), *Phonological intervention: Concepts and procedures* (pp. 13–34). San Diego: College-Hill Press.

Folkins, J. W., & Bleile, K. M. (1990). Taxonomies in biology, phonetics, phonology and speech motor control. *Journal of Speech and Hearing Disorders, 55,* 596–611.

Foster, R., Giddan, J., & Stark, J. (1972). *Assessment of children's language comprehension.* Palo Alto, CA: Consulting Psychologists Press.

Fowler, C. A., & Turvey, M. (1980). Immediate compensation in bite-block speech. *Phonetica, 37,* 306–326.

Frisch, G., & Handler, L. (1974). A neuropsychological investigation of functional disorders of speech articulation *Journal of Speech and Hearing Research, 17,* 432–445.

Galaburda, A. M., & Eidelberg, D. (1982). Symmetry and asymmetry in the human posterior thalamus, II: Thalamic lesions in a case of developmental dyslexia. *Archives of Neurology, 39,* 333–336.

Galaburda, A. M., & Kemper, T. L. (1979). Cytoarchitectonic abnormalities in developmental dyslexia: A case study. *Annals of Neurology, 6,* 94–100.

Galaburda, A. M., LeMay, M., Kemper, T. L., & Geschwind, N. (1978). Right-left asymmetries in the brain. *Science, 199,* 852–856.

Galaburda, A. M., Sherman, G. F., Rosen, G. D., Aboitz, F., & Geschwind, N. (1985). Developmental dyslexia: Four consecutive patients with cortical anomalies. *Annals of Neurology, 18,* 222–233.

Garn-Nunn, P., & Martin, V. (1992). Using conventional tests with highly unintelligible children: Identification and programming concerns. *Language, Speech, and Hearing Services in Schools, 23,* 52–60.

Garvey, M., & Mutton, D. (1973). Sex chromosome aberrations and speech development. *Archives of Disease in Childhood, 48,* 937–941.

Gay, T., Lindblom, B., & Lubker, J. (1981). Production of bite-block vowels: Acoustic equivalence by selective compensation. *Journal of the Acoustical Society of America, 69,* 802–810.

Geschwind, N. (1975). The apraxias: Neural mechanisms of disorders of learned movement. *American Scientist, 63,* 188–195.

Geschwind, N. (1979). Anatomical foundation of language and dominance. In C. Ludlow & M. E. Doran-Quine (Eds.), *The neurological bases of language disorders in children: Methods and directions for research* (pp. 145–157) (NINCDS Monograph 22). Washington, DC: Government Printing Office.

Geschwind, N., & Behan, P. (1982). Left-handedness: Association with immune disease, migraine, and developmental learning disorder. *Proceedings of the National Academy of Science USA, 79,* 5097–5100.

Geschwind, N., & Levitsky, W. (1968). Human brain right-left asymmetries in temporal speech region. *Science, 161,* 186–187.

Glasson, C. (1981, November). *Spectrographic analysis of developmental apraxia: Temporal coordination difficulties.* Presentation at the American Speech-Language-Hearing Association Convention, Los Angeles.

Glasson, C. (1984). Speech timing in children with history of phonological-phonetic disorders. *Seminars in Speech and Language, 5,* 85–95.

Goldman, R., & Fristoe, M. (1986). *Goldman-Fristoe test of articulation.* Circle Pines, MN: American Guidance Service.

Gubbay, S. (1978). The management of developmental apraxia. *Developmental Medicine and Child Neurology, 20,* 643–646.

Guyette, T., & Diedrich, W. (1981). A critical review of developmental apraxia of speech. In N. Lass (Ed), *Speech and language: Advances in basic research and practice* (Vol. 5, pp. 1–49). New York: Academic Press.

Hall, P., Hardy, J., & LaVelle, W. (1990). A child with signs of developmental apraxia of speech with whom a palatal lift prosthesis was used to manage palatal dysfunction. *Journal of Speech and Hearing Disorders, 55,* 454–460.

Haslam, R., Dalby, J. T., Johns, R.D., & Rademaker, A. W. (1981). Cerebral asymmetry in developmental dyslexia. *Archives of Neurology, 38,* 679–682.

Hecaen, H. (1976). Acquired aphasia in children and the ontogenesis of hemispheric functional specialization. *Brain and Language, 3,* 114–134.

Hecaen, H., & Albert, M. (1978). *Human neuropsychology.* New York: John Wiley.

Heilman, K. M., Schwartz, H. D., & Geschwind, N. (1975). Defective motor learning in ideomotor apraxia. *Neurology, 25,* 1018–1020.

Helfrich-Miller, K. (1984). Melodic intonation therapy with developmentally apraxic children. *Seminars in Speech and Language, 5,* 119–126.

Hier, D. B., LeMay, M., Rosenberger, P. B., & Perlo, V. P. (1978). Developmental dyslexia: Evidence for a subgroup with a reversal of cerebral asymmetry. *Archives of Neurology, 35,* 90–92.

Hodson, B. (1980). *The assessment of phonological processes.* Danville, IL: Interstate Printers and Publishers.

Hughes, M., & Sussman, H. M. (1983). An assessment of cerebral dominance in language-disordered children via a time-sharing paradigm. *Brain and Language, 19,* 48–64.

Huttenlocher, P. R. (1979). Synaptic density in human frontal cortex: Developmental changes and effects of aging. *Brain Research, 163,* 195–205.

Ingram, D. (1976). *Phonological disability in children.* London: Edward Arnold.

Jackson, J. H. (1878/1932). Remarks on non-protrusion of the tongue in some cases of aphasia. In J. Taylor, *Selected writings of John Hughlings Jackson* (Vol. 2). London: Hodder & Stoughton.

Jaffe, M. B. (1984). Neurologic impairment of speech production: Assessment and treatment. In J. Costello (Ed.), *Speech disorders in children: Recent advances* (pp. 157–186). San Diego: College-Hill Press.

Kahneman, D. (1973). *Attention and effort.* Englewood Cliffs, NJ: Prentice-Hall.

Kelso, J. A. S., & Tuller, B. (1983). "Compensatory articulation" under conditions of reduced afferent information: A dynamic formulation. *Journal of Speech and Hearing Research, 26,* 217–224.

Kemper, T. (1982). Asymmetrical lesions in dyslexia. Paper presented at the course on *Biological Foundations of Cerebral Dominance*. Boston, MA: Harvard University.

Kent, R., Kent, J., & Rosenbek, J. (1987). Maximum performance tests of speech production. *Journal of Speech and Hearing Disorders, 52,* 367–387.

Kent, R. D., & McNeil, M. R. (1987). Relative timing of sentence repetition in apraxia of speech and conduction aphasia. In J.H. Ryalls (Ed.), *Phonetic approaches to speech production in aphasia and related disorders* (pp. 181–220). San Diego: College-Hill Press.

Kimura, D. (1976). The neural basis of language qua gesture. In H. Whitaker & H. A. Whitaker (Eds.), *Studies in neurolinguistics* (Vol. 2, pp. 145–156). New York: Academic Press.

Kimura, S. (1978). Acquisition of a motor skill after left hemisphere damage. *Brain, 100,* 527–542.

Kimura, D., & Watson, N. (1989). The relation between oral movement control and speech. *Brain and Language, 37,* 565–590.

Kinsbourne, M., & McMurray, J. (1975). The effect of cerebral dominance on time sharing between speaking and tapping by preschool children. *Child Development, 46,* 240–242.

Kirk, S., McCarthy, J., & Kirk, W. (1968). *Illinois test of psycholinguistic abilities.* Urbana, IL: University of Illinois Press.

Ladefoged, P. (1975). *A course in phonetics.* New York: Harcourt Brace Jovanovich.

Lahey, M. (1990). Who shall be called language disordered? Some reflections and one perspective. *Journal of Speech and Hearing Disorders, 55,* 612–620.

Landau, W. M., Goldstein, R., & Kleffner, F. R. (1960). Congenital aphasia: A clinicopathologic study. *Neurology, 10,* 915–921.

LaPointe, L. L., & Erickson, R. J. (1991). Auditory vigilance during divided task attention in aphasic individuals. *Aphasiology, 5,* 511–520.

LaPointe, L., & Wertz, R. T. (1974). Oral-movement abilities and articulatory characteristics of brain-injured adults. *Perceptual Motor Skills, 39,* 39–46.

Lee, L. (1969). *The Northwestern syntax screening test.* Evanston, IL: Northwestern University Press.

Lee, L. (1974). *Developmental sentence analysis.* Evanston, IL: Northwestern University Press.

LeMay, M. (1977). Asymmetries of the skull and handedness: Phrenology revisited. *Journal of Neurological Sciences, 32,* 243–253.

Lenneberg, E. H. (1967). *Biological foundations of language.* New York: John Wiley.

Liles, B. L. (1975). *An introduction to linguistics.* Englewood Cliffs, NJ: Prentice-Hall.

Locke, J. L. (1983). Clinical phonology: The explanation and treatment of speech sound disorders. *Journal of Speech and Hearing Disorders, 48,* 339–341.

Lou, H.C., Henriksen, L., & Bruhn, P. (1984). Focal cerebral hypoperfusion in children with dysphasia and/or attention deficit disorder. *Archives of Neurology, 41,* 825–829.

Ludwig, C. (1983). *An interaction study of phonology and length of utterance in developmental verbal dyspraxics and normals in repetition and conversational speech.* Unpublished doctoral dissertation, Southern Illinois University, Carbondale.

Ludwig, C., & Crary, M. A. (1981). *Influence of performance load on phonological profiles obtained in developmental verbal dyspraxia subjects.* Unpublished manuscript. Southern Illinois University, Carbondale.

Luria, A. R. (1980). *Higher cortical functions in man.* New York: Basic Books. (Original work published in 1962)

Malinsky, A. E. (1985). *Syngery: A therapy approach for developmental verbal dyspraxia.* Unpublished master's thesis, Southern Illinois University, Carbondale.

Margolin, D. I. (1984). The neuropsychology of writing and spelling: Semantic, phonological, motor, and perceptual processes. *The Quarterly Journal of Experimental Psychology, 36A,* 459–489.

Marquardt, T., & Sussman, H. (1984). The elusive lesion-apraxia of speech link in Broca's aphasia. In J. Rosenbek, M. McNeil, & A. Aronson (Eds.). *Apraxia of speech: Physiology, acoustics, linguistics, management* (pp. 91–112). San Diego, CA: College-Hill Press.

Marquardt. T., & Sussman, H. (1991). Developmental apraxia of speech: Theory and practice. In D. Vogel & M. Cannito (Eds.), *Treating disordered speech motor control* (pp. 341–390). Austin, TX: Pro-Ed.

Marshall, J. L., & Newcombe, F. (1973). Patterns of paralexia: A psycholinguistic approach. *Journal of Psycholinguistic Research, 2,* 175–197.

Mason, S. M., & Mellor, D. H. (1984). Brain-stem, middle latency and late cortical evoked potentials in children with speech and language disorders. *Electroencephalography and Clinical Neurophysiology, 59,* 297–309.

Mateer, C. (1978). Impairments of nonverbal oral movements after left hemisphere damage: A follow-up analysis of errors. *Brain and Language, 6,* 334–341.

Mateer, C. (1983). Motor and perceptual functions of the left hemisphere and their interaction. In S. J. Segalowitz (Ed.), *Language functions and brain organization* (pp. 145–170). New York: Academic Press.

Mateer, C., & Kimura, D. (1977). Impairment of nonverbal oral movements in aphasia. *Brain and Language, 4,* 262–276.

McCarthy, R., & Warrington, E. K. (1984). A two-route model of speech production: Evidence from aphasia. *Brain, 107,* 463–485.

McDonald, E. (1964). *Articulation testing and treatment: A sensory motor approach.* Pittsburgh: Stanwix House.

McNeil, M. R., Odell, K., & Tseng, C. H. (1991). Toward the integration of resource allocation into a general theory of aphasia. In T. Prescott (Ed.), *Clinical aphasiology* (Vol. 20, pp. 21–39). Austin, TX: Pro-Ed.

Mecham, J., Jex, J., & Jones, J. (1967). *Utah test of language development* (rev. ed.). Salt Lake City, UT: Communication Research Association.

Miller, J. F. (1981). *Assessing language production in children.* Baltimore: University Park Press.

Mlcoch, A. G., & Noll, J. D. (1980). Speech production models as related to the concept of apraxia of speech. In N. J. Lass (Ed.), *Speech and language: Advances in basic research and practice* (pp. 201–237). New York: Academic Press.

Morley, M. (1965). *The development and disorders of speech in childhood.* Baltimore: Williams & Wilkins.

Morley, M., Court, D., & Miller, H. (1954). Developmental dysarthria. *British Medical Journal, 1,* 8–10.

Morley, M., Court, D., Miller, H., & Garside, R. (1955). Delayed speech and developmental aphasia. *British Medical Journal, 2*, 463–467.

Nathan, P. W. (1947). Facial apraxia and apraxic dysarthria. *Brain, 70*, 449–478.

Nebes, R. (1975). The nature of inner speech in a patient with aphemia. *Brain and Language, 2*, 489–497.

Netsell, R. (1985). Construction and use of a bite-block for the evaluation and treatment of speech disorders. *Journal of Speech and Hearing Disorders, 50*, 103–106.

Ojemann, G., & Mateer, C. (1979). Cortical and subcortical organization of human communication: Evidence from stimulation studies. In H. Steklis & M. Raleigh (Eds.), *The neurobiology of social communication in primates* (pp. 111–131). New York: Academic Press.

Palmer, M., Wuth, C., & Kincheloe, J. (1964). The incidence of lingual apraxia and agnosia in "functional" disorders of articulation. *Cerebral Palsy Review, 25*, 7–9.

Pannbacker, M. (1988). Management strategies for developmental apraxia of speech: A review of the literature. *Journal of Communication Disorders, 21*, 363–371.

Parkins, R. A., Roberts, R. J., Reinarz, S. J., & Varney, N. R. (1987, February). *CT asymmetries in adult developmental dyslexics.* Paper presented to the International Neuropsychological Society, Washington, DC.

Patton, M., Baraister, M., & Brett, M. (1986). A family with congenital suprabulbar paresis (Worster-Drought syndrome). *Clinical Genetics, 29*, 147–150.

Peters, A. M. (1977). Language learning strategies: Does the whole equal the sum of the parts? *Language, 53*, 560–573.

Piazza, D. M. (1977). Cerebral lateralization in young children as measured by dichotic listening and finger tapping tasks. *Neuropsychologia, 15*, 417–425.

Plante, E. (1991). MRI findings in the parents and siblings of specifically language-impaired boys. *Brain and Language, 41*, 67–80.

Plante, E., Swisher, L. Vance, R., & Rapcsak, S. (1991). MRI findings in boys with specific language impairment. *Brain and Language, 41*, 52–66.

Poliakov, G. I. (1961). Some results of research into the development of the neuronal structure of the cortical ends of the analyzers in man. *Journal of Comparative Neurology, 117*, 197–212.

Raade, A., Rothi, L., & Heilman, K. (1991). The relationship between buccofacial and limb apraxia. *Brain and Cognition, 16*, 130–146.

Rakic, R., Bourgeois, J. P., Eckenhoff, M.R., Zecevic, N., & Goldman-Rakic, P. S. (1986). Concurrent overproduction of synapses in diverse regions of the primate cerebral cortex. *Science, 232*, 232–235.

Rapin, I., & Allen, D. A. (1983). Developmental language disorders: Nosologic considerations. In U. Kirk (Ed.) *Neuropsychology of language, reading and spelling* (pp. 213–219). New York: Academic Press.

Ratcliffe, S. (1982) Speech and learning disorders in children with sex chromosome abnormalities. *Developmental Medicine and Child Neurology, 24*, 80–84.

Ratcliff, G., Dila, C., Taylor, L., & Milner, B. (1980). The morphological asymmetry of the hemispheres and cerebral dominance for speech: A possible relationship. *Brain and Language, 11*, 87–98.

Risser, A., & Edgell, D. (1988). Neuropsychology of the developing brain: Implication for neuropsychological assessment. In M. Tramontana & S. Hooper (Eds.), *Assessment issues in child neuropsychology* (pp. 41–66). New York: Plenum.

Robinson, R. (1991). Causes and associations of severe and persistent specific speech and language disorders in children. *Developmental Medicine and Child Neurology, 33*, 943–962.

Rosenbek, J., Hansen, R., Baughman, C., & Lemme, M. (1974). Treatment of developmental apraxia of speech: A case study. *Language, Speech and Hearing Services in Schools, 5*, 13–22.

Rosenbek, J., & Wertz, R. T. (1972). A review of 50 cases of developmental apraxia of speech. *Language, Speech and Hearing Services in Schools, 3*, 23–33.

Roy, E. (1978). Apraxia: A new look at an old syndrome. *Journal of Human Movement Studies, 4*, 191–210.

Roy, E. A., & Square, P. (1985). Common considerations in the study of limb, verbal, and oral apraxia. In E. A. Roy (Ed.), *Neuropsychological studies of apraxia and related disorders* (pp. 111–161). North Amsterdam: Elsevier Science.

Saleeby, N., Hadjian, S., Martinkosky, S., & Swift, M. (1978, November). *Familial verbal dyspraxia: A clinical study*. Presentation to the American Speech-Language-Hearing Association Convention, San Francisco.

Satz, P., & Bullard-Bates, C. (1981). Acquired aphasia in children. In M. T. Sarno (Ed.), *Acquired aphasia* (pp. 399–426). New York: Academic Press.

Schumacher, J., McNeil, M. R., & Yoder, D. (1984). *Efficacy of treatment: Melodic intonation therapy with developmentally apraxic children*. Presentation to the American Speech-Language-Hearing Association Convention, San Francisco.

Shallice, T., & Warrington, E.K. (1975). Word recognition in a phonemic dyslexic patient. *The Quarterly Journal of Experimental Psychology, 27*, 187–199.

Shelton, R. L., & McReynolds, L. V. (1979). Functional articulation disorders: Preliminaries to treatment. In N. Lass (Ed.), *Speech and language: Advances in basic research and practice* (Vol. 2, pp. 1–111). New York: Academic Press.

Shriberg, L., & Kwiatkowski, J. (1980). *Natural process analysis*. New York: John Wiley.

Shriberg, L., & Kwiatkowski, J. (1988). A follow-up study of children with phonologic disorders of unknown origin. *Journal of Speech and Hearing Disorders, 53*, 144–155.

Simonds, R. J., & Schiebel, A. B. (1989). The postnatal development of the motor speech area: A preliminary study. *Brain and Language, 37*, 42–58.

Snowling, M., & Stackhouse, J. (1983). Spelling performance of children with developmental verbal dyspraxia. *Developmental Medicine and Child Neurology, 25*, 430–437.

Sparks, R., Helm, N., & Albert, M. (1974). Aphasia rehabilitation resulting from melodic intonation therapy. *Cortex, 10*, 303–316.

Sparks, R., & Holland, A. (1976). Method: Melodic intonation therapy for aphasia. *Journal of Speech and Hearing Disorders, 41*, 284–297.

Spriestersbach, D. C., Morris, H., & Darley, F. (1978). Examination of the speech mechanism. In F. Darley & D. C. Spriestersbach (Eds.), *Diagnostic methods in speech pathology* (2nd ed.), (pp. 322–345). New York: Harper & Row.

Stark, R. (1985). Dysarthria in children. In J. Darby (Ed.), *Speech and language evaluation in neurology: Childhood disorders* (pp. 185–217). Orlando, FL: Grune & Stratton.

Stark, R., & Tallal, P. (1981). Selection of children with specific language deficits. *Journal of Speech and Hearing Disorders, 46*, 114–122.

Stinchfield, S., & Young, R. (1938). *Children with delayed and defective speech: Motor-kinesthetic factors and their training*. Palo Alto, CA: Stanford University Press.

Sussman, H., Marquardt, T., Hutchinson, J., & MacNeilage, P. (1986). Compensatory articulation in Broca's aphasia. *Brain and Language, 27*, 56–74.

Tallal, P., & Piercy, M. (1974). Developmental aphasia: rate of auditory processing and selective impairment of consonant perception. *Neuropsychologia, 12,* 83–93.

Tallal, P., & Piercy, M. (1975). Developmental aphasia: the perception of brief vowels and extended stop consonants. *Neuropsychologia, 13,* 69–74.

Tallal, P., & Stark, R. (1976). Relation between speech perception and speech production impairment in children with developmental dysphasia. *Brain and Language, 3,* 305–317.

Tallal, P., Stark, R., Kallman, C., & Mellits, D. (1980). Developmental dysphasia: Relation between acoustic processing deficits and verbal processing. *Neuropsychologia, 18,* 273–284.

Tallal, P., Townsend, J., Curtiss, S., & Wulfeck, B. (1991). Phenotypic profiles of language-impaired children based on genetic/family history. *Brain and Language, 41,* 81–95.

Tallman, V., & Crary, M. A. (1985, November). *Production of propositional prosody by children with developmental verbal dyspraxia.* Presentation to the American Speech-Language-Hearing Association Convention, Washington, DC.

Templin, M., & Darley, F. (1960). *The Templin-Darley tests of articulation.* Iowa City: University of Iowa Bureau of Educational Research and Service.

Tognola, G., & Vignolo, L. A. (1980). Brain lesions associated with oral apraxia in stroke patients: A clinico-neuroradiological investigation with the CT scan. *Neuropsychologia, 18,* 257–272.

Tompkins, C. A., & Flowers, C. R. (1985). Perception of emotional intonation by brain-damaged adults: The influence of task processing level. *Journal of Speech and Hearing Research, 28,* 527–538.

Towne, R., & Melgren, L. (1987, November). *Lingual-mandibular dependency and diadochokinesis in children.* Presentation to the American Speech-Language-Hearing Association Convention, New Orleans.

Van Riper, C. (1972) *Speech correction: Principles and methods.* Englewood Cliffs, NJ: Prentice-Hall.

VanDongen, H. R., Loonen, M. C. B., & VanDongen, K. J. (1985). Anatomical basis for acquired fluent aphasia in children. *Annals of Neurology, 17,* 306–309.

Wada, J. A., Clarke, R., & Hamm, A. (1975). Cerebral hemispheric asymmetry in humans. *Archives of Neurology, 32,* 239–246.

Weckler, A., & Crary, M. A. (1982). *Developmental verbal dyspraxia: A therapy study.* Presentation to the American Speech-Language-Hearing Association Convention, Toronto.

Weeks, T. (1974). *The slow speech development of a bright child.* Lexington, MA: D. C. Heath.

Weitz, R., Varsano, I., Geifman, M., Grunebaum, M., & Nitzan, M. (1976). Cricopharyngeal achalasia associated with congenital suprabulbar paresis. *Helv. paediat. Acta, 31,* 271–274.

Wertz, R. T. (1985). Neuropathologies of speech and language: An introduction to patient management. In D. F. Johns (Ed.), *Clinical management of neurogenic communication disorders* (pp. 1–96). Boston: Little, Brown.

Whitaker, H. A. (1971). Neurolinguistics. In W. Dingwall (Ed.), *A survey of linguistic science* (pp. 137–251). College Park, MD: University of Maryland Press.

Williams, R., Ingham, R., & Rosenthal, J. (1981). A further analysis for developmental apraxia of speech in children with defective articulation. *Journal of Speech and Hearing Research, 24,* 496–505.

Witelson, S. F., & Pallie, W. (1973). Left hemisphere specialization for language in the newborn. *Brain, 96,* 641–646.

Wolff, P. H., Michel, G. F., & Ovrut, M. (1990). The timing of syllable repetitions in developmental dyslexia. *Journal of Speech and Hearing Research, 33,* 281–289.

Worster-Drought, C. (1953). Failure in normal language development of neurological origin. *Folia Phoniatrica, 5,* 130–145.

Worster-Drought, C. (1956). Congenital suprabulbar paresis. *The Journal of Laryngology and Otology, 70,* 453–463.

Worster-Drought, C. (1974). Suprabulbar paresis: Congenital suprabulbar paresis and its differential diagnosis with special reference to acquired suprabulbar paresis. *Developmental Medicine and Child Neurology, 16*(Suppl. 30), 1–33.

Yakovlev, P. I., & Lecours, A. R. (1967). The myelogenetic cycles of regional maturation of the brain. In A. Minkowski (Ed.), *Regional development of the brain in early life* (pp. 3–70). Oxford: Blackwell.

Yorkston, K., Beukelman, D., & Bell, K. (1988). *Clinical management of dysarthric speakers.* San Diego: College-Hill Press.

Yoss, K., & Darley, F. (1974a). Developmental apraxia of speech in children with defective articulation. *Journal of Speech and Hearing Research, 17,* 399–416.

Yoss, K., & Darley, F. (1974b). Therapy in developmental apraxia of speech. *Language, Speech and Hearing Services in Schools, 5,* 23–31.

Young, E., & Hawk, S. (1955). *Moto-kinesthetic speech training.* Palo Alto, CA: Stanford University Press.

Zaidel, E. (1979). The split and half brain as models of congenital language disability. In C. L. Ludlow & M. E. Doran-Quine (Eds.), *The neurological basis of language disorders in children: Methods and directions for research* (pp. 55–89). NINCDS Monograph 22. Washington, DC: Government Printing Office.

Zaidel, E. (1985). Language in the right hemisphere. In D. F. Benson & E. Zaidel (Eds.), *The dual brain: Hemispheric specialization in humans* (pp. 205–231). New York: Guilford Press.

Zlatin, M., & Koenigsknecht, R. (1976). Development of the voicing contrast: A comparison of voice onset time in stop perception and production. *Journal of Speech and Hearing Research, 19,* 93–111.

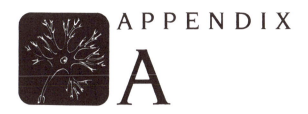

APPENDIX A

Example of a Background Questionnaire for Child Patients

Background Information Questionnaire

Identification Information

Child's Name: Date:

Address: D.O.B.:

Phone: Age:

Parent/Guardian: Sex: M F

Referral Source:

Area of Concern

Please describe your concern regarding your child's speech, language, and/or hearing:

When did you first become aware of this difficulty?

Is your child aware of any difficulty/difference in the way he/she speaks (or aware of a hearing problem)?

Developmental History

Birth History:

   Mother's age at time of birth:

   Accidents/illnesses during pregnancy:

   Medication taken during pregnancy (specify):

   Length of pregnancy:

   Delivery/Perinatal Complications?

When did your child first (age in months):

   Sit Up:

   Crawl:

   Walk:

   Feed Self:

   Dress Self:

   Toilet Trained: Day: Night:

   Please describe any problems or concerns with any of the listed areas.

Medical History

Has your child had the following diseases? When? What treatment was used?

   Mumps:

   Measles:

   Scarlet Fever:

   Chicken Pox:

   Croup:

   Ear Infections (How often?):

   Upper Respiratory Infections (How often?):

   Other:

Does your child have a persisting medical condition that we should be aware of?

Has your child had any serious accidents (specify)?

Is your child presently on medication (specify)?

Has your child had any surgery (specify)?

Speech and Language Development

Did your child babble before speaking his/her first words? (Describe)

How old was your child when first words were spoken? (What were they?)

When did your child begin to put words together?

Does (or did) your child use gestures to communicate? (with speech? instead of speech?)

When did your child first begin to put two words together?

When did your child first begin to speak in sentences?

Does your child us "baby talk"?

Is your child easily understood?

   By family members:

   By persons outside the immediate family:

Have there been any abrupt changes in your child's manner of speaking?

Has your child ever received speech/language therapy? (Please provide details.)

Do you have any reason to suspect that your child may have a hearing problem?

Social/Family History

Father's Occupation:

Mother's Occupation:

How many children in the family? (Please specify sex and age.)

Does your child get along with:

Family members:

Outside peers:

Does your child interact better with children or adults?

Please list a few things your child likes/dislikes to do.

Does anyone else in your family have a speech, language, or hearing problem?

Educational History

When did your child start school?

What grade is he/she currently enrolled in?

Does he/she have any problems in school?

Is he/she in a special classroom?

Has he/she ever repeated a grade (which)?

Does your child like school?

Comments

Is there any information you would like to add that might aid us in working with your child?

B

Operational Definitions of 13 Phonological Processes Used with the Phonological Process Analysis Described in Chapter 8

Clinical Assessment of Phonological Processes
Michael A. Crary, Ph.D.
(Revised June 1982)

In an attempt to simplify and operationalize an approach to phonological process analyses, commonly reported processes have been selected and organized into a clinically applicable system. A major focus of this system is to quantify the results of descriptive linguistic analysis. Toward this goal, a group of processes has been defined to increase the reliability of their identification and to provide some quantifiable structure to this assessment approach. Using these definitions, a series of investigations was completed to evaluate variables influencing phonological process analysis such as sample size, percent of errors accounted for, and intra- and interjudge reliability. The following pages present the operational definitions of this group of processes.

Initially, 13 processes were included in the analysis. These were divided into two groups: (a) six basic processes that are commonly seen in both normal and disordered speakers—and—which are common intervention targets, and (b) an additional seven processes which have been useful in describing phonological profiles in severely disordered children and adults. It is important to note that this system is not intended to replace a basic knowledge of phonological process analysis. Rather, it is designed for use by clinicians possessing some skills in the area but who are searching for a more quantifiable technique within the approach.

The Basic Six

1. Deletion of Final Consonants (DFC)

   a. General Description: Omission of syllable final consonants or consonant clusters.

   b. Specific Errors:

CVC → CV	kæt → kæ
CVC CVC → CV CV	bæθtʌb → bætʌ
CVCC → CV	gost → go

2. Cluster Reduction (CR)

   a. General Description: Reduction or alternation of any prevocalic consonant cluster.

   b. Specific Errors:

Type 1: $C_1C_2VC_3 \rightarrow C_1VC_3$	trʌk → tʌk
Type 2: $C_1C_2VC_3 \rightarrow C_1C_4VC_3$	trʌk → twʌk
Type 3: $C_1C_2VC_3 \rightarrow C_4VC_3$	trʌk → dʌk
Type 4: $C_1C_2VC_3 \rightarrow C_4C_5VC_3$	trʌk → dwʌk

   Note: If the entire initial cluster is omitted count the error as DIC and make a parenthetical note under CR to indicate that the omission involved a cluster.

   Note: Final cluster errors, with the exception of omission of the entire cluster, are noted parenthetically under CR; however, these are not counted in the numerical analysis. When the entire final cluster is omitted, count as DFC but not the error parenthetically under CR.

3. Stopping (ST)

   a. General Description: Replacement of a fricative or affricate with a stop.

b. Specific Errors:

s,θ → t	tʃ → t,k
z,ð → d	dʒ → d,g
f → p	
v → b	
ʃ → t,k	
ʒ → d,g	

Note: Children may "stop liquids" or other sound classes (e.g., l → d). When observed these errors should be noted parenthetically under ST but counted in a separate analysis.

4. Gliding (GL)

a. General Description: Replacement of a liquid with a glide.

b. Specific Errors:

r → w,j
l → w,j

Note: Children may "glide" other sound classes (e.g., fricatives). When observed these errors should be parenthetically noted under GL but counted as a separate analysis.

5. Fronting (FR)

a. General Description: Production of a velar or palatal sound at an al-veolar place of articulation.

b. Specific Errors:

k → t	tʃ → t,ts	ʒ → z
g → d	dʒ → d,dz	ʃ → s

Note: If a sound is "fronted" by replacement by a labial do *not* count as FR. This is counted as "labialization." Substitution of s → θ or similar patterns should *not* be counted as FR. These are counted as "lisping" or "stridency deletion."

Note: If the velar nasal /ŋ/ is fronted to /n/ as part of a secondary stress applied to the -ing ending do *not* count as an error.

6. Backing (BK)

a. General Description: Production of an alveolar or labial sound at a more posterior (palatal or velar) place of articulation.

b. Specific Errors:

p,t → k	s → ʃ	m,n → ŋ,g
b,d → g		

Note: Productions of /ʔ/ or /h/ for oral consonants should *not* be counted as BK. These errors are counted as glottal replacement. (When a /ʔ/ re-places an oral consonant at the end of a syllable count the error as DFC.)

An Additional Seven

7. Deletion of Initial Consonants (DIC)

   a. General Description: Omission of any syllable initial consonant or consonant cluster.

   b. Specific Errors:

CVC → VC	kæt → æt
CVC CVC → VC VC	bæθtʌb → æʔʌb
CCVC → VC	stap → ap

   Note: When an entire initial cluster is omitted note the error parenthetically under CR as well as counting it as DIC. If an oral consonant is replaced by /h/ in the prevocalic position count as glottal replacement.

8. Glottal Replacement (GR)

   a. General Description:
      (1) Replacement of oral consonants with /ʔ/ or /h/.
      (2) Omission of intervocalic consonants even if a /ʔ/ is not perceived.

   Note: The first category does not apply to syllable final consonants.

9. Weak Syllable Deletion (WSD)

   a. General Description: Omission of any syllable not receiving primary stress in polysyllabic words.

10. Prevocalic Voicing (PVV)

    a. General Description: A voiceless obstruent becomes voiced before a vowel (syllable initial position).

    Note: This does not apply to intervocalic (ambisyllabic) consonants.

11. Vocalization (VOC)

    a. General Description: Replacement of a syllabic consonant, final /r/ or /l/, or vocalic /ʒ/ or /ʃ/ with a full vowel.

    b. Specific Errors:

l̩ → o	CVr → CVʊ	ʒ̩, ʃ → o,a,ə,ʊ
r̩ → ʊ,ə,ɑ	CVl → CVo	
m̩ → ʊ		
n̩ → ʊ		

12. Vowel Neutralization (VN)

    a. General Description: Vowels are produced as /a/ or /ə/.

    Note: This does not include syllabic consonants nor /ʒ/ or /ʃ/ (see VOC).

13. Labialization (LAB)

    a. General Description: Replacement of any lingual consonant with a labial consonant.

Note: This process has been observed so infrequently in our disordered subjects that is now considered in the "Other" category. In some cases it may be *the* dominant process, but this is rare.

Other Phonological Processes

Twelve of the 13 phonological processes listed in the preceding pages are seen frequently in children with severe speech disorders. They are not the only error patterns we have observed; but they are the most prevalent and the "strongest." Following is a listing of other phonological processes that have been noted with some frequency or which may be strong for individual children. Descriptions of these errors may be found in literature concerning phonological process analysis.

1. Labialization (see 13 above)
2. Apicalization
3. Voicing alterations (other than PVV)
4. Nasality alterations
5. Lisping or specific stridency deletion
6. Specific phonetic markers

Multiple Processes

Although the processes have been presented individually, it is entirely possible that more than one process will operate on a given production or erred segment. If the processes cannot be identified it is advised that the clinician note the error in distinctive feature terminology and specify the position of the syllable where occurred. The same strategy should be followed for infrequent or unusual errors. It is important to remember that this system is not intended to replace a basic knowledge of phonological principles or, more specifically, of phonological process analyses. This system is designed to expedite analyses for clinicians possessing the appropriate basic knowledge.

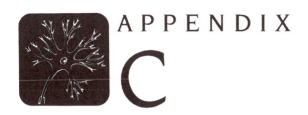

APPENDIX

C

60-Phrase Imitation Procedure Used in Studies of Phonological Performance in Children with Developmental Apraxia of Speech

Phrases for Phonological Analysis

1983 (Revised)

M. A. Crary

Department of Communicative Disorders
J. Hillis Miller Health Center
University of Florida
Gainesville, FL 32610

Target	Transcription
1. Get the *hammer*.	
2. Use the *comb*.	
3. Cut with a *knife*.	
4. It's a *penny*.	
5. Buy the *ring*.	
6. Chase the *pig*.	
7. Read the *paper*.	
8. In the *tub*.	
9. Buy the *coffee*.	
10. In the *van*.	
11. At the *movies*.	
12. That's a *badger*.	
13. Eat the *fudge*.	
14. At the *zoo*.	
15. Wear the *shirt*.	
16. Hold the *cup*.	
17. Eat the *cookie*.	
18. See the *duck*.	
19. Hold the *baby*.	

Target	Transcription
20. Climb the *ladder*.	
21. Shoot the *gun*.	
22. Push the *wagon*.	
23. Hit the *ball*.	
24. Eat the *carrot*.	
25. It is *yellow*.	
26. On the *stove*.	
27. Hurt my *thumb*.	
28. In my *mouth*.	
29. Give me *that*.	
30. Pick the *feathers*.	
31. It's so *smooth*.	
32. On the *chair*.	
33. Light the *matches*.	
34. Check your *watch*.	
35. Near the *sun*.	
36. Hold the *glasses*.	
37. In the *house*.	
38. It's a *zebra*.	
39. Use the *scissors*.	
40. Tie my *shoe*.	
41. Wash the *dishes*.	
42. Catch the *fish*.	
43. Brush my *teeth*.	

Target	Transcription
44. Ride the *train*.	
45. Get the *toy*.	
46. Milk the *cow*.	
47. Shoot the *bird*.	
48. Eat the *cracker*.	
49. Open the *jar*.	
50. Ride the *plane*.	
51. Hop like a *frog*.	
52. He is a *prince*.	
53. Eat the *grape*.	
54. A funny *clown*.	
55. Take a *drink*.	
56. She's a *twin*.	
57. Eat with a *spoon*.	
58. Put on the *skates*.	
59. She's a *queen*.	
60. Catch the *snake*.	

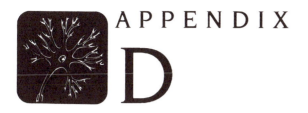

D

Analysis Form for Phonological Process Analysis from the 60-Phrase Imitation Procedure

Please note that the transcriptions are presented in simple format. Clinicians should recognize regional variants in production, especially those associated with vowels and stress patterns.

PHONOLOGICAL PROCESSES

TARGET	RESPONSE	SYLLABLE SHAPE	ERRORS (-)->(-)	DFC	DIC	CR	WSD	GR	ST	GL	FR	BK	PVV	LAB	VOC	VOW. NEUT.	OTHER
1. hæmən																	
2. kom																	
3. narf																	
4. peni																	
5. rɪg																	
6. pig																	
7. pepən																	
8. tʌb																	
9. kɔfi																	
10. væn																	
11. muviz																	
12. bɔdʒən																	
13. fʌdʒ																	
14. zu																	
15. ʃɜt																	
16. kʌp																	
17. kʌki																	

PHONOLOGICAL PROCESSES

TARGET	RESPONSE	SYLLABLE SHAPE	ERRORS (-)->(-)	DFC	DIC	CR	WSD	GR	ST	GL	FR	BK	PVV	LAB	VOC	VOW. NEUT.	OTHER
18. dʌk																	
19. bebɪ																	
20. lædə																	
21. gʌn																	
22. wægən																	
23. bɔl																	
24. kɛrɪt																	
25. jɛlo																	
26. stov																	
27. θʌm																	
28. mʌv⊖																	
29. dɑrt																	
30. fɛðəz																	
31. smʌʤ																	
32. tʃɛr																	
33. mæʧɪz																	
34. wɑtʃ																	

PHONOLOGICAL PROCESSES

TARGET RESPONSE SYLLABLE ERRORS

SYLLABLE: SHAPE

ERRORS: (-) -> (-)

TARGET	RESPONSE	SYLLABLE SHAPE	ERRORS (-)→(-)	DFC	DIC	CR	WSD	GR	ST	GL	FR	BK	PVV	LAB	VOC	VOW. NEUT.	OTHER
35. sʌn																	
36. glæsɪz																	
37. havs																	
38. zibrə																	
39. sizənz																	
40. ʃu																	
41. dɪʃɪz																	
42. fɪʃ																	
43. ti·θ																	
44. tren																	
45. tɔɪ																	
46. kav																	
47. bɜd																	
48. kræker																	
49. dʒar																	
50. plen																	
51. frɔg																	

PHONOLOGICAL PROCESSES

TARGET	RESPONSE	SYLLABLE SHAPE	ERRORS (-)->(-)	DFC	DIC	CR	WSD	GR	ST	GL	FR	BK	PVV	LAB	VOC	VOW. NEUT.	OTHER
52. Prints																	
53. grep																	
54. klarn																	
55. dribk																	
56. twin																	
57. spun																	
58. skets																	
59. kwin																	
60. snek																	
			Total # occur:														
			Total # Potential:	44	60	17	16	61	37	4	26	64	22	—	12	50	1
			RS value (% error)														

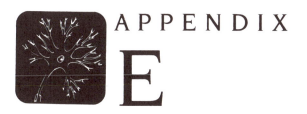

Sample of a Completed Phonological Process Analysis

Blanks in the response column indicate acceptable productions. Numbers in parentheses in the "CR" column indicate the type of cluster reduction as presented in Appendix B.

PHONOLOGICAL PROCESSES

TARGET	RESPONSE	SYLLABLE SHAPE	ERRORS (–)→(–)	DFC	DIC	CR	WSD	GR	ST	GL	FR	BK	PVV	LAB	VOC	NEUT.	OTHER
1. hæmɚ	hæmʊ		ɚ→ʊ												ɚ		
2. kɔm	tɔ:	-m	k→t	m							k						
3. naɪf	na:	-f	aɪ→a	f												aɪ	
4. pɛnɪ																	
5. rɪŋ	wɪŋ		r→w							r							
6. pɪg	pɪ	-g		g													
7. pɛpɚ	pɛpʊ		ɚ→ʊ												ɚ		
8. tʌb																	
9. kʌtʃɪ	tʌtʃɪ		k→t								k						
10. vɛn	bɛn		v→b						v								
11. muviz	muvi	-z		z													
12. bæʤɚ	bæʤʊ		ɚ→ʊ, ʤ→d						dʒ						ɚ		
13. fʌʤz	fʌd		ʤ→d						dʒ								
14. zu	du		z→d						N								
15. ʃɚt	tʊt		ʃ→t, ɚ→ʊ						s						ɚ		
16. kʌp	tʌʔ	-p	k→t	p							k						
17. kʊkɪ	tʊtɪ		k→t, k→t								k						

TARGET   RESPONSE   SYLLABLE   ERRORS

PHONOLOGICAL PROCESSES

SHAPE   (-)→(-)

TARGET	RESPONSE	SYLLABLE SHAPE	ERRORS (-)→(-)	DFC	DIC	CR	WSD	GR	ST	GL	FR	BK	PVV	LAB	VOC	NEUT.	OTHER
18. dʌk	dʌʔ	-k		k													
19. bebɪ																	
20. lædɚ	wædɚ	-h	l→w, ɚ→v							l					ɚ		
21. gʌn	gʌ	-h		n													
22. wægən	wædʌn	-l	g→d								g						
23. bɔl	ba:	-l	ɔ→a	l						l						ɔ	
24. kɛrɪt	tɛwI	-t	k→t, r→w	t						r	k						
25. jɛlo																	
26. stov	to:v	st→t				st (?)											
27. θʌm																	
28. mʌv θ	mavt	-t	θ→t						⊖								
29. dɔt	dɔʔ	-t	d→d	t					ð								
30. fɛdɚz	fɛdɚz	-z	d→d, ɚ→v	z		sm (?)			ð						ɚ		
31. smʌʧ	mʌʧ	sm→s															
32. ʧɛr	tɛ	-r	ʧ→t	r					ʧ								
33. mɔtʰɪz	mɔtʰɪz	-z	ʧ→t	z					ʧ								
34. waʧ	wat		ʧ→t	t					ʧ								

PHONOLOGICAL PROCESSES

TARGET	RESPONSE	SYLLABLE SHAPE	ERRORS (-)→(-)	DFC	DIC	CR	WSD	GR	ST	GL	FR	BK	PVV	LAB	VOC	VOW. NEUT.	OTHER
35. sʌn	tʌn		s→t	z		sl(1)			ˈs								
36. glæsɪz	gætɪ	gl→g -z	s→t	s					s								
37. hɑrs	hɑr	-s															
38. zibrə	dibə	br→b	z→d	z		br(1)		z						ɚ			
39. sɪzɚz	titʊ	-z	s→t, z→ʔ ɚ→ʊ	z				z	s								
40. ʃu	du		s→d	s					s	ʃ——s							
41. dɪʃɪz	dɪtɪ	-z	s→t	z					s	ʃ——s							
42. fɪʃ	fɪ	-ʃ		ʃ													
43. tiθ																	
44. trɛn	twɛn		tr→tw			tr(2)											
45. tɔɪ																	
46. kɑʊ																	
47. bɝd	bʊd	-r	ʃ→v												ɝ		
48. krækɚ	tæʔʊ	kr→t	k→ʔ ɚ→ʊ			kr(3)	k								ɚ		
49. dʒɑr	dɑ	-r	dʒ→z	r													
50. plɛn	pɛn	pl→p				pl(1)											Fric.
51. frɔg	fwɑ:	-g	fr→fw	g		fr(2)											

PHONOLOGICAL PROCESSES

VOW.

TARGET	RESPONSE	SYLLABLE SHAPE	ERRORS (-)->(-)	DFC	DIC	CR	WSD	GR	ST	GL	FR	BK	PVV	LAB	VOC	NEUT.	OTHER
S2. prints	PI:	-nts / pr->p	nts	pr (1)													
S3. grep	gwep	gr->gw		gr (2)													
S4. klwrn	+avrn	kl->t		kl (3)													
S5. dribk	dwI:	-bk	bk	gr (2)													
S6. twin																	
S7. spun	puh	sp->p		sp (1)													
S8. skets	tet	sk->t (ts->t)		sk (3)													
S9. kwin	twin	kw->tw		kw (2)													
60. snek	nek	sn->n		sn (1)													
		Total # occur:	nts 22	-	16	1	2	16	3	10	-	1	1	8	2	1	
		Total # Potential:	44	60	17	16	61	37	4	26	64	22	-	12	50	1	
		RS value (% error)	.50		.94	.03	.43	.75	.39			.05		.67	.04		

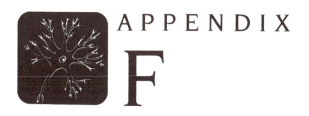

APPENDIX F

A Multifocal Intervention Approach for Cases of Developmental Motor Speech Disorders

Sample Therapy Program for Open/Closed Syllable Shapes

Specific Goals

1. To increase proportion of closed (CVC) syllable shapes in conversational speech.
2. To increase production of plural and possessive grammatical morphemes in conversational speech.

General Procedure

Each 40–50 minute therapy session will include a three phase program incorporating the following:

1. Oral motor/phonetic tasks
2. Phonemic contrasting of open (CV) and closed (CVC) syllables. Initial closed targets (CVC) will be primarily nasals and fricatives.
3. Incorporation of targeted minimal word pairs into syntactic units. Specific grammatical morphemes include plural and possessive markers /s/ and /z/, and auxiliaries /ɪz/ and /ar/ plus present progressive verbs.

Phase I: Oral Motor/Phonetic

A bite block is placed between the first molars to stabilize the mandible. With the block in place the child will produce (attempt) each of the following sounds and sound sequences three times in succession:

/i/a/u/   /ia/ua/iu/   /iju/awi/ju/wi/   /digu/gidu/tiku/kitu/

Example:

After the bite block has been placed between upper and lower molars, the clinician will model sounds and ask the child to repeat three times.

Clinician: "I'm going to say some sounds and I want you to say the same sound. I'm going to ask you to say them more than once. Ready? Say /i/."

Child: "/i/"

Clinician: "Good, now say it again."

Child: "/i/"

Clinician: "Great, now one more time."

Child: "/i/"

Clinician: "Super, now say /a/," etc.

The goal of this procedure is not correct production of target sounds, but rather anterior, posterior, high and low independent tongue movement. If the child needs the model repeated, the clinician should do so as often as necessary. Recommended time for phase I is 5–10 minutes. As performance improves, lengthen strings of phonetic targets and increase complexity of syllable shapes to CVC.

Phase II: Phonemic Contrasting

Using minimal word pairs (depicted as pictures on cards) for CV/CVC syllable shapes, a phonemic contrasting method will be utilized including the following steps:

1. *Modeling*

The clinician will present minimal word pairs one card at a time and identify the picture. Each word will then be established as either an open word

(CV) or a closed word (CVC). Distinction between the members of each pair will be made with visual cues and verbal descriptions of mouth positions at the end of the words. The clinician will then put the card into the correct pocket of the word board (a large piece of cardboard or cloth with three pockets: one containing all cards and one for each member of the contrast).

Example:

Clinician: "This is a bee. Bee is an open word. Bee is open because my mouth stays open at the end. I'm putting the bee into the open pocket. This is a bean. Bean is a closed word. Bean is closed because my tongue closes my mouth in the front. I'm putting bean into the closed pocket," and so on. (The actual metaphors used to describe the contrast are best selected in reference to the child's language and conceptual abilities.)

All words are presented one at a time in this manner; however, the word pairs are emphasized as a unit. It is important that the child understand all words used as minimal pairs. Some changes in the word list may be necessary.

2. *Discrimination*
The clinician presents paired word cards. Each card is named individually and the child is asked to indicate the correct picture and determine whether that word is open or closed. Cards are placed into correct pockets on the word board by the child. The clinician should continue reinforcement of the CV/CVC distinction with visual and verbal cues. Any child who is unable to discriminate between the two syllable shapes should receive additional work in this area.

3. *Imitation*
Paired cards are presented in the same manner as step 2. The child is asked to repeat each target production before indicating the correct card and identifying words as either open or closed. Incorrect productions (i.e., CV productions for CVC targets) should be identified as open words. Continued description of closed word production is important. Initially closure with any lingual or labial sound is accepted as correct. The clinician may ask for repeat attempts but the major focus should be stimulation and not drilling.

Example:

Clinician: "This is a bee. What is this?"

Child: "A bee."

Clinician: "Right. Is bee an open word or a closed word?"

Child: "Closed?"

Clinician: "Listen and watch me as I say the word. Bee. Is my mouth open or do I close it with my tongue?"

Child: "It stays open."

Clinician: "Right. Bee is an open word because my mouth stays open at the end. Now, this is a bean. What is this?"

Child: "A bee."

Clinician: "I'm listening very carefully and I'm watching your mouth. You left your mouth open at the end of that word. Bee is an open word. Listen and watch me as I say this word. Bean. My tongue closed that word at the front of my mouth. Try this one again."

Child: "beat."

Clinician: "Great, you closed that word. When you say bean your tongue closes your mouth," and so on.

Cards are placed into correct pockets and another word pair is chosen.

4. *Production*

Paired cards are presented and the child is asked to be the teacher. The child produces one of the words and the clinician chooses a card. Both cards in each pair should be attempted before presenting the next pair. Initially, it is probable that the CVC word will be produced as a CV word. Although the clinician may be aware that intended production was CVC, response should depend on production. When such errors are made, stimulation for closed words should continue. Again, drilling is not necessary and all closures should be accepted.

Example:

Clinician: "Now I want you to be the teacher. You say a word and I'll pick the one you say."

Child: "Bee."

Clinician: "This is a bee. You left your mouth open and bee is an open word. Am I right? Okay, your turn again."

Child: "Bee."

Clinician: "Bee. (attempt to reproduce child's production). You left your mouth open at the end of that word. Bee is an open word. Is this the right one?"
(points to bee)

Child: "No, no I mean beat."

Clinician: "Oh, you closed the word that time. Bean is a closed word. Is this the right one?"
(points to bean)

Cards are then placed in the correct pocket and the next word pair is presented.

5. *Performance Load Building*

Child or clinician chooses one or two pair cards and tells a story or makes up a sentence using both words. Clinician may need to ask child to repeat a sentence initially but spontaneous use is the goal of this step.

Note: The number and type of minimal word pairs chosen is dependent on the individual child. Five word pairs are recommended as a starting point. A good idea is to use some words the child is known to produce correctly as a built-in success motivator in the early sessions. Replacing word pairs on a regular basis often fends off boredom. Recommended time for phase II is 20 minutes.

Phase III: Syntactice Expression

Using selected word pairs from phase II, the Fokes Sentence Builder, and spontaneous dialogue, the clinician and child will develop syntactic units with emphasis on the following: plural and possessive markers /s/ and /z/, auxiliary plus present progressive verbs and copula plus descriptors. Suggested time is 10 minutes.

Example:

The boy is running./The boys are running.

A play period of approximately 10 minutes is recommended for communicative interaction at the end of each session.

An Alternative Format for Phonemic Contrasting

The phonemic contrasting approach presented above is somewhat dry and tutorial. Fokes (1982) recommends a more pragmatic, interactive approach to phonemic contrasting. Consider the following conversation facilitating a front-back contrast described by Fokes (1982, p. 29).

The clinician presents the appropriate pictures as the session progresses.

Child picks up a picture.

Child	*Clinician*
	Yes, a car. And this is a picture of tar. The tar is gooey, and the tar is on the car. Remember to move your tongue to the front of your mouth and say "tar."
/ka:/	
	What did you say? Did you say "car?" Say "tar."

Child	Clinician
/ta:/	
	Yes, tar. Tar is on the car.
/ta:/ . . . /ka:/	
	Now, here is Dee. She has a key to the car. What does she have?
/ki/	
	A key. Who has the key?
/ki/	
	Who? Not "key" but "Dee." Move your tongue to the front of your mouth. Say "Dee."
/di/ /di/ have a /ki/. a /ki/ in the /ka:/	
	And what does the car have on it?
/ka:/ have /ka:/	
	The car has what on it?
/ta:/ on /ka:/	

The clinician presents all word pairs in a similar manner
until the deck of words is completed.

	Now, let's tell our story. This is a story about Dee. Dee has a key to a car. Dee has a key.
/di/ have /ki/	
	Dee is riding down the road in her car. The car is full of tar. Tar is on her car.
/ka:/ on /ka:/	
	What? What is on the car? Tar?
/ta:/ in on the /ka:/	
	A gust of wind blew on the car. Now the car is full of dust. A gust of wind blew dust on the car.
/gʌ/ of wind. It blow /dʌ/.	
	Dee saw Kurt down the road. Kurt said, "Look at the dirt on the car." Kurt pointed to the dirt.
/kʊ:/ point to /dʊ:/ /ka:/ have /ta:/ too	
	Yes, it's full of goo, too. It's gooey.
/ka:/ /gui/ /tu/	
	Dee said, "I must take care of my car. I don't want to tear up my car. I don't want to . . . . . ."
. . . . . .	
	I don't want to tear up my car.
/tɛ/ up, /tɛ/ /ka:/	

Child	Clinician
	Yes, Dee wants to take care of her car.
/ke ke/	
	Take care.
/te ke, te ke/	
	Take care of the car.
/te ke/ of /kaː/	
	Who? Who is taking care of the car?
/gi/	
	Who? What's her name?
/gi/ . . . /di/	
	Yes, Dee. Dee has a car. And Dee has a key.

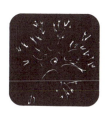

Index